WHO Technical Report Series

855

EVALUATION OF CERTAIN VETERINARY DRUG RESIDUES IN FOOD

Forty-third report of the
Joint FAO/WHO Expert Committee on
Food Additives

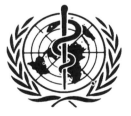

World Health Organization

Geneva 1995

WHO Library Cataloguing in Publication Data

Joint FAO/WHO Expert Committee on Food Additives
    Evaluation of certain veterinary drug residues in food :
    forty-third report of the Joint FAO/WHO Expert Committee
    on Food Additives.

    (WHO technical report series ; 855)

    1. Food contamination 2. Drug residues – analysis
    3. Drug therapy – veterinary   I. Title II. Series

    ISBN 92 4 120855 4   (NLM Classification: WA 701)
    ISSN 0512-3054

Printed in Switzerland
95/10521 – Benteli – 7500

Contents

Joint FAO/WHO Expert Committee on Food Additives

Geneva, 15–24 November 1994

Members

Dr F. A. Abiola, Director, Interstate School of Veterinary Sciences and Medicine, Dakar, Senegal

Dr L.-E. Appelgren, Professor of Pharmacology, Department of Pharmacology and Toxicology, Faculty of Veterinary Medicine, The Swedish University of Agricultural Sciences, Biomedical Centre, Uppsala, Sweden

Dr D. Arnold, Director, Centre for Surveillance and Health Evaluation of Environmental Chemicals, Berlin, Germany (*Joint Rapporteur*)

Dr J. Boisseau, Director, Laboratory of Veterinary Drugs, National Centre of Veterinary and Food Studies, Fougères, France (*Vice-Chairman*)

Dr L. Cuerpo, Senior Researcher, Meat Technology Department, National Institute of Agricultural Technology, Research Centre of Veterinary Sciences, Buenos Aires, Argentina

Dr R. Ellis, Director, Chemistry Division, Food Safety and Inspection Service, Department of Agriculture, Washington, DC, USA (*Joint Rapporteur*)

Dr R. D. Furrow, Beltsville, MD, USA

Dr J. D. MacNeil, Head, Food Animal Chemical Residues Section, Health of Animals Laboratory, Agriculture and Agri-Food Canada, Saskatoon, Saskatchewan, Canada

Professor J. G. McLean, Pro Vice-Chancellor, Division of Science, Engineering and Design, Swinburne University of Technology, Hawthorn, Victoria, Australia (*Chairman*)

Dr A. Pintér, Deputy Director-General, National Institute of Hygiene, Budapest, Hungary

Professor A. Rico, Biochemistry–Toxicology, Physiopathology and Experimental Toxicology Laboratory (INRA), National Veterinary School, Toulouse, France

Dr P. Sinhaseni, Associate Professor, Department of Pharmacology, Faculty of Pharmaceutical Sciences, Chulalongkorn University, Bangkok, Thailand

Dr R. Wells, Director, Research and Development, Australian Government Analytical Laboratories, Pymble, New South Wales, Australia

Dr K. Woodward, Director of Licensing, Veterinary Medicines Directorate, Ministry of Agriculture, Fisheries and Food, New Haw, Addlestone, Surrey, England

Dr M. Yndestad, Professor of Food Hygiene, Department of Food Hygiene, Norwegian College of Veterinary Medicine, Oslo, Norway

Secretariat

Dr C. E. Cerniglia, Director, Division of Microbiology, National Center for Toxicological Research, Jefferson, AR, USA (*WHO Temporary Adviser*)

Dr P. Chamberlain, Veterinary Medical Officer, Center for Veterinary Medicine, Food and Drug Administration, Rockville, MD, USA (*WHO Consultant*)

Dr R. Fuchs, Deputy Minister, Ministry of Sciences, Zagreb, Croatia (*WHO Temporary Adviser*)

Dr L. Gajjar, Formerly at Veterinary Medicines Directorate, Ministry of Agriculture, Fisheries and Food, New Haw, Addlestone, Surrey, England (*WHO Temporary Adviser*)

Dr R. J. Heitzman, Science Consultant, Newbury, Berkshire, England (*FAO Consultant*)

Dr J. L. Herrman, Scientist, International Programme on Chemical Safety, WHO, Geneva, Switzerland (*Joint Secretary*)

Dr A. R. M. Kidd, Independent Veterinary Consultant, Woking, Surrey, England (*WHO Temporary Adviser*)

Dr R. C. Livingston, Director, Office of New Animal Drug Evaluation, Center for Veterinary Medicine, Food and Drug Administration, Rockville, MD, USA (*FAO Consultant*)

Dr K. Mitsumori, Chief, Third Section, Division of Pathology, Biological Safety Research Centre, National Institute of Hygienic Sciences, Tokyo, Japan (*WHO Temporary Adviser*)

Dr L.T. Mulligan, Office of New Animal Drug Evaluation, Center for Veterinary Medicine, Food and Drug Administration, Rockville, MD, USA (*WHO Temporary Adviser*)

Dr J. Paakkanen, Food Control Officer, Food Quality Liaison Group, Food Quality and Standards Service, Food and Nutrition Division, FAO, Rome, Italy (*Joint Secretary*)

Dr L. Ritter, Executive Director, Canadian Network of Toxicology Centres, University of Guelph, Guelph, Ontario, Canada (*WHO Temporary Adviser*)

Dr G. Roberts, Director, Toxicology Evaluation Section, Department of Human Sciences and Health, Canberra, Australia (*WHO Temporary Adviser*)

Dr B. Röstel-Peters, Secretary, Committee for Veterinary Medicinal Products Working Group on Safety of Residues, Directorate-General III/E/3, Pharmaceuticals, Commission of the European Communities, Brussels, Belgium (*WHO Temporary Adviser*)

Dr S. Sundlof, Director, Center for Veterinary Medicine, Food and Drug Administration, Rockville, MD, USA (*WHO Temporary Adviser*)

Dr F. X. R. van Leeuwen, Senior Toxicologist, Toxicology Advisory Centre, National Institute of Public Health and Environmental Protection, Bilthoven, Netherlands (*WHO Temporary Adviser*)

Monographs containing summaries of relevant data and toxicological evaluations are available from WHO under the title:

Toxicological evaluation of certain veterinary drug residues in food. WHO Food Additives Series, No. 34, 1995.

Residues monographs are issued separately by FAO under the title:

Residues of some veterinary drugs in animals and foods. FAO Food and Nutrition Paper, No. 41/7, in press.

INTERNATIONAL PROGRAMME ON CHEMICAL SAFETY

The preparatory work for toxicological evaluations of food additives and contaminants by the Joint FAO/WHO Expert Committee on Food Additives (JECFA) is actively supported by certain of the Member States that contribute to the work of the International Programme on Chemical Safety (IPCS).

The International Programme on Chemical Safety (IPCS) is a joint venture of the United Nations Environment Programme, the International Labour Organisation, and the World Health Organization. One of the main objectives of the IPCS is to carry out and disseminate evaluations of the effects of chemicals on human health and the quality of the environment.

1. Introduction

A meeting of the Joint FAO/WHO Expert Committee on Food Additives was held at WHO headquarters, Geneva, from 15 to 24 November 1994. The meeting was opened by Dr M. Mercier, Director of the International Programme on Chemical Safety, on behalf of the Directors-General of the Food and Agriculture Organization of the United Nations and the World Health Organization.

Dr Mercier noted that many of the veterinary drugs that would be considered at the meeting had a long history of use. As requested by the Committee at its fortieth meeting, manufacturers should provide evaluation reports on such substances when data meeting current standards are not available; otherwise Acceptable Daily Intakes (ADIs) and Maximum Residue Limits (MRLs) cannot be established. Dr Mercier also noted that the assessment of microbiological risk resulting from residues of antimicrobial drugs is very difficult because of the lack of validated procedures for estimating the risk, and he hoped that further progress could be made at the present meeting. Further studies will be needed, and clear recommendations to governments and/or industry for further work should enable advances to be made in this area.

The six previous meetings of the Committee to consider veterinary drug residues in food (Annex 1, references *80, 85, 91, 97, 104,* and *110*) had been held in response to the recommendations of the Joint FAO/WHO Expert Consultation held in 1984 (*1*). The present meeting[1] was convened in response to the recommendation made at the forty-second meeting of the Committee that meetings on this subject should be held annually (Annex 1, reference *110*). The Committee's purpose was to provide guidance to FAO and WHO Member States and to the Codex Alimentarius Commission on public health issues pertaining to residues of veterinary drugs in foods of animal origin. The specific tasks before the Committee were:

(a) to elaborate further principles for evaluating the safety of residues of veterinary drugs in food and for establishing ADIs and MRLs for such residues when the drugs under consideration are administered to food-producing animals in accordance with good practice in the use of veterinary drugs (see section 2);

(b) to evaluate the safety of residues of certain veterinary drugs (see section 3 and Annexes 2 and 3); and

(c) to discuss matters of interest arising from the report of the Eighth Session of the Codex Committee on Residues of Veterinary Drugs in Foods (*2*).

---

[1] As a result of the recommendations of the first Joint FAO/WHO Conference on Food Additives held in 1955 (FAO Nutrition Meeting Report Series, No. 11, 1956; WHO Technical Report Series, No. 107, 1956), there have been 42 previous meetings of the Joint FAO/WHO Expert Committee on Food Additives (Annex 1).

2. General considerations

2.1 Principles governing the safety evaluation of residues of veterinary drugs in food

In making recommendations on the safety of residues of veterinary drugs in food, the Committee took into consideration the principles contained in *Principles for the safety assessment of food additives and contaminants in food* (Annex 1, reference *76*), in the thirty-second, thirty-fourth, thirty-sixth, thirty-eighth, fortieth, and forty-second reports of the Committee (Annex 1, references *80, 85, 91, 97, 104,* and *110*) and in the report of the Joint FAO/WHO Expert Consultation on Residues of Veterinary Drugs in Food (*1*).

2.2 Modification of the agenda

Apramycin, imidocarb and ractopamine were removed from the agenda because information for their review was not provided.

Enrofloxacin and azaperone were added to the agenda for both toxicological and residues evaluation and dexamethasone was added for residues evaluation.

2.3 Evaluation of veterinary drugs with a long history of use

The Codex Committee on Residues of Veterinary Drugs in Foods has established criteria for selecting compounds for inclusion on its list of substances proposed for evaluation by the Joint FAO/WHO Expert Committee on Food Additives (*2, 3*). From the Expert Committee's deliberations on a variety of veterinary products that meet the Codex Committee's criteria, it has been apparent that, for certain products with a long history of use, toxicological or chemical residue data have been provided that do not meet modern standards for analysis, but none the less may be useful in the safety assessment of residues in human food. Accordingly, at its fortieth meeting (Annex 1, reference *104*), the Expert Committee developed a scientifically acceptable approach for evaluating the safety of these products. However, at its present meeting, the Committee recognized that there may be some difficulty in identifying drugs that qualify for evaluation using this approach.

The Committee identified some typical examples of situations where products might be considered as drugs having a long history of use. A drug may have been originally developed as a human therapeutic agent, but later been used as a veterinary drug in single or companion animals and finally in food-producing animals. This evolution of veterinary use may have occurred over more than a decade with the use in food-producing animals emerging relatively recently. Examples of products in this category include β-agonists and tranquillizers. Data may be inadequate for drugs with a long history of use where no sponsor has exclusive commercial rights to a product and where a veterinary drug was registered before requirements for toxicological and residue data were established (in many countries, around 1980) by drug registration authorities.

The Committee recognized that for veterinary drugs with a long history of use, the toxicological data were likely to have been generated in the early stages of drug development and would, therefore, be assessed by the Committee on the basis of guidelines described in its fortieth report (Annex 1, reference *104*). However, when a new use for such a drug was proposed, the Committee expected that new data would be generated according to modern protocols for toxicological and residue studies. The Committee noted, for example, that residue data originally submitted for the evaluation of residues in food-producing animals may have contained, as a minimum, data on metabolism and depletion and information on methods of analysis for residues. Where a new use was being proposed, more comprehensive residue data would be required, including data on total residues obtained in radiometric studies and information on bound residues.

The Committee recommended that, if it is desired that a veterinary drug be evaluated under the procedures described in the report of its fortieth meeting for a veterinary drug with a long history of use, this should be stipulated by the sponsor when the dossier is submitted. The Committee, however, reserves the right to decide which substances qualify as drugs with a long history of use.

The Committee recognized that individual sponsors are often reluctant to generate data for veterinary drugs for which they do not have exclusive commercial rights. Nevertheless, the Committee requires adequate data to establish an ADI and to recommend appropriate MRLs. The Committee encourages the establishment of consortia to provide the necessary resources to generate the required data. Groups that might be considered include drug sponsors, government agencies and manufacturers' groups or associations.

2.4 Veterinary drugs identified for priority consideration

Most of the veterinary drugs that are reviewed by the Committee are originally placed on the agenda because they have been identified as drugs requiring priority attention by the Codex Committee on Residues of Veterinary Drugs in Foods. To be placed on the priority list of the Codex Committee, a veterinary drug must satisfy several criteria. One criterion has been that the sponsor must undertake to provide a dossier on the compound for review by the Expert Committee. However, the Codex Committee criteria have been revised recently (*2*), and the submission of a dossier is no longer an absolute requirement.

Nevertheless, even when submission of data was required, substances have sometimes had to be removed from the agenda, because dossiers were not available. This occurred again at the present meeting and delays consideration of other drugs of equal priority on which data could have been supplied.

Clearly, the Expert Committee cannot evaluate substances without adequate data being made available for review in a timely manner. The Expert Committee therefore supports efforts to develop more effective procedures to ensure that adequate dossiers will be available on substances that are placed on the priority list. There is a strong need for a joint commitment by the Secretariat of the Expert Committee, the Codex Committee and a sponsor or consortium (see section 2.3) to generate the necessary data. The Committee stressed the necessity for drug sponsors to provide in a timely fashion all relevant available information on veterinary drugs addressing the end-points of concern.

2.5 Veterinary drugs used in aquaculture

Veterinary drugs are used in aquaculture in finned fish, eels, molluscs and crustacea. Such use may result in residues of these veterinary drugs being present in the edible tissues of these species. The Committee therefore recognized the need for establishing some general guidelines for the safety evaluation of drug residues resulting from aquaculture production.

2.5.1 *Consumption*

The human consumption of farmed fish and prawns, for example, seems to vary considerably and accurate food intake data are difficult to obtain at the international level. In order to protect all segments of the population, MRLs for these food commodities should be based on the food intake values noted in the thirty-fourth report of the Committee (Annex 1, reference *85*), although this report does not specifically refer to food items produced by aquaculture. In the European Union, MRLs for fish are based on a daily intake of 300 grams of muscle and skin in natural proportions (*4*). This food intake value is the same as that used by the thirty-fourth Committee for recommending MRLs in muscle tissue of food-producing animals and should be considered as an alternative to meat consumption. The Committee agreed that this is an appropriate value to use for recommending MRLs for veterinary drugs used in aquaculture.

2.5.2 *Residue analysis in aquaculture*

In its review of certain veterinary drugs used in aquaculture, the Committee noted that during treatment with drugs such as oxolinic acid, flumequine and oxytetracycline, there are high concentrations of residues of these drugs in the skin of fish. Because the rate of depletion of veterinary drugs from muscle is generally more rapid than from skin, the concentration of drug residues in skin may be higher than in the corresponding muscle at the recommended withdrawal period. The Committee recognized that muscle is the main edible tissue in fish, but that it is often consumed in combination with skin in natural proportions. Therefore, when analysing farmed fish for residues of veterinary drugs, analyses should be carried out on samples of muscle and skin in natural proportions. The size of the samples should be large enough so that the contribution of residues from the skin and muscle tissue is representative of the whole fish.

The Committee did not have sufficient data on residues of veterinary drugs in food items produced by aquaculture. The Committee recommended, as an interim measure, to use for residue analysis only those tissues that are normally consumed. In addition, the Committee requested information from national authorities on procedures used for the control of residues of veterinary drugs in food produced by aquaculture.

3. Comments on residues of specific veterinary drugs

The Committee evaluated for the first time the safety and residues of four antimicrobial agents. It re-evaluated the safety and residues of one β-adrenoceptor-blocking agent, three antimicrobial agents and one tranquillizing agent, and the residues of one glucocorticosteroid. The recommendations made with regard to these compounds are given in Annex 2, while details of further toxicological studies and other information required or desired are given in Annex 3.

Toxicological monographs or monograph addenda were prepared on all the substances considered in this section, except oxolinic acid and dexamethasone. Residues monographs or monograph addenda were prepared on all the substances.

References are provided in the toxicological assessment of oxolinic acid in this report because a toxicological monograph was not prepared, which would normally contain such references.

3.1 β-Adrenoceptor-blocking agent

3.1.1 *Carazolol*

Carazolol is a nonspecific β-adrenoceptor-blocking agent, primarily used in pigs to prevent sudden death due to stress during transport. It had previously been evaluated at the thirty-eighth meeting of the Committee (Annex 1, reference 97), when a temporary ADI of 0–0.1 µg per kg of body weight was established. At that time, additional data were requested concerning the pharmacological no-effect level in humans, which were provided for the present meeting.

Toxicological data

The Committee considered results from clinical trials in healthy human volunteers and in patients suffering from sympatheticotonia, hypertension, angina pectoris, cardiac arrhythmia, chronic bronchitis or asthma. Because pharmacological effects were observed at all dose levels, no-effect levels were derived from these results by extrapolation. For this purpose, a linear relationship was assumed between the observed pharmacological effects and the logarithm of the administered dose. The Committee noted that this approach resulted in a conservative estimate of the no-effect levels.

Several of the studies that were submitted were considered to be inadequate for the calculation of a no-effect level, owing to the absence of a clear dose–effect relationship or because only a single dose level was used.

In an ergometric exercise test in 12 healthy human volunteers, the effect on cardiac function was determined following administration of a single oral dose of 5 or 7.5 mg of carazolol per person. From the dose–response curve, a no-effect level of 10 µg per kg of body weight was extrapolated.

Patients suffering from either chronic bronchitis or asthma showed reductions in vital capacity and forced expiratory volume 2 hours after administration of a single oral dose of 0.1 or 0.7 mg of carazolol per person (5 individuals per dose group). Based on these results, corrected for the apparent differences in the starting values of both parameters between the two dose groups, the overall no-effect level was 0.5 µg per kg of body weight.

The Committee recognized that humans with chronic bronchitis or asthma are highly sensitive to the effects of carazolol. It also recognized that this subgroup forms a substantial part of the general population and that adequate allowance should be made for variation between individuals.

The Committee noted that the previous temporary ADI of 0–0.1 µg per kg of body weight provided a margin of safety of 100 in relation to the no-effect level of 10 µg per kg of body weight derived from data in healthy volunteers. It also noted that the no-effect level of 0.5 µg per kg of body weight derived from studies in highly sensitive individuals suffering from chronic bronchitis or asthma provided a margin of safety of 5. The Committee concluded that these values provided adequate allowance for variation between individuals and therefore established an ADI of 0–0.1 µg per kg of body weight.

Residue data

At its thirty-eighth meeting, the Committee had reviewed the results of various residue-depletion studies on carazolol:

- a radiometric study of the pharmacokinetics and excretion of carazolol in pigs;
- two pharmacokinetic studies in cattle;
- metabolism studies in pigs, dogs and humans;
- two radiometric residue-depletion studies in pigs;
- two residue-depletion studies in pigs; and
- a residue-depletion study in cattle.

The Committee had also reviewed information on a high-performance liquid chromatography (HPLC) method of analysis.

At the thirty-eighth meeting, the Committee recommended temporary MRLs for carazolol of 5 µg/kg for muscle and fat and 30 µg/kg for liver and kidney in both cattle and pigs and requested the results of the following studies for evaluation:

1. Radiometric studies on the concentrations of carazolol and its metabolites as proportions of the total residue in pigs and cattle over a 24-hour period.
2. Nonradiometric studies on carazolol residues in pigs, using suitable analytical methods, over a 24-hour period.

No new data were submitted for cattle at the present meeting. However, results were available from a nonradiometric residue-depletion study in which carazolol was administered by intramuscular injection in the neck at a dose of 10 µg per kg of body weight to 16 pigs. Groups of four animals were slaughtered at 2, 12, 18 and 24 hours after injection, and samples of muscle, kidney, fat, liver, skin and tissue at the injection site were taken for determination of carazolol by HPLC with fluorometric detection and a limit of quantification of 2 µg/kg of tissue. The limits of detection were approximately 0.2 µg/kg for muscle, kidney and skin, 0.7 µg/kg for liver, and 0.6 µg/kg for fat. The residues at 2 hours after injection were 56.8, 1.8, 6.9, 9.9, 1.8 and 2.5 µg/kg in the injection site, muscle, kidney, liver, fat and skin, respectively. Carazolol was depleted rapidly from all tissues and all samples were at the limit of quantification at 12 hours after dosing. Residues in muscle and fat were at the limit of detection at 12 hours after injection.

Maximum Residue Limits

At its present meeting, the Committee noted that the metabolites/residues other than carazolol have been demonstrated not to contribute significantly to the β-adrenoceptor-blocking activity of the residues. Based on the ADI of 0–0.1 µg/kg for parent carazolol established by the Committee, the permitted daily intake is 6 µg for a 60-kg person.

The Committee established MRLs for carazolol based on the concentrations determined at 2 hours after administration in the HPLC study in pigs, which were 1.8 µg/kg for muscle, 9.9 µg/kg for liver, 6.9 µg/kg for kidney, and 1.8 µg/kg for fat. It concluded that the residue concentrations would be below the MRLs when the drug is used according to the approved conditions of use. Using the concentrations of carazolol determined by HPLC at 2 hours after dosing and adding at least three statistical standard deviations, the Committee recommended MRLs in pigs of 5 µg/kg for muscle and fat/skin, and 25 µg/kg for liver and kidney, expressed as parent drug. These MRLs would result in a daily maximum intake of 5.5 µg of carazolol, based on a daily food intake of 300 g of muscle, 100 g of liver, and 50 g each of kidney and fat.

The Committee did not recommend MRLs for cattle.

The issue of the safety of the injection site is of particular importance for drugs such as carazolol that have no or very short withdrawal periods. The main residue at the injection site is likely to be parent drug; in the HPLC residue study the average concentration of carazolol at 2 hours after injection was 56.8 µg/kg.

The Committee noted that the concentration of residues of carazolol at the injection site 2–4 hours after injection was in the range 30–100 µg/kg. If 300 g of muscle tissue was ingested from this site, this could result in consumption of 30 µg of carazolol, well in excess of the maximum ADI of 6 µg per day, which was based on the acute pharmacological effects of carazolol. The Committee recommended that registration authorities should pay particular attention to the potential risk of residues of carazolol in tissue at the injection site. Considering the potential risk, the Committee concluded that the use of carazolol in pigs to reduce stress during transport to slaughter is inconsistent with the safe use of veterinary drugs in food-producing animals.

3.2 Antimicrobial agents

The Committee examined the results of *in vitro* antimicrobial activity studies using relevant human gut microflora to calculate ADIs for some of the antimicrobial agents that were reviewed. The equation used for deriving these ADIs is based on Annex 5 of the report of the thirty-eighth meeting of the Committee (Annex 1, reference *97*), in which an equation was provided for the derivation of temporary ADIs. At its forty-second meeting (Annex 1, reference *110*), the Committee concluded that this approach could also be used for the establishment of final ADIs.

The upper limit of the ADI is derived as follows:

$$\text{Upper limit of ADI (µg/kg of body weight)} = \frac{\text{Concentration without effect on human gut flora (µg/ml)} \times \text{Daily faecal bolus (g)}}{\text{Fraction of oral dose bioavailable} \times \text{Safety factor} \times \text{Weight of human (60 kg)}}$$

The *concentration without effect on human gut flora,* the *fraction of oral dose bioavailable,* and the *safety factor* may vary, depending upon the circumstances relating to the particular veterinary drug under consideration. The reasons for using particular factors are given in the individual evaluations.

The average weight of the daily faecal bolus is known to vary widely among individuals from 150 g to over 400 g per day; in addition, drug concentrations in the rectum are greater than in the more proximal portions of the colon. In estimating the ADIs in this report, the Committee adopted a very conservative approach, assuming the average weight of the daily faecal bolus was 150 g.

3.2.1 *Dihydrostreptomycin and streptomycin*

Both dihydrostreptomycin and streptomycin were previously evaluated at the twelfth meeting of the Committee (Annex 1, reference *17*). An ADI was not established for either compound at that time.

The two compounds are aminoglycoside antibiotics, and are closely related in structure. They are used for treatment of bacterial infections in food-producing animals.

Dihydrostreptomycin is formed by reduction of streptomycin. The pharmacokinetic properties, toxicological profile, and spectrum of antimicrobial and biological activity of the two compounds are similar. Therefore, data on the two compounds were considered together for the purpose of establishing a single ADI. The Committee noted that the two compounds are generally considered together in the published literature, including the report of its twelfth meeting.

Toxicological and microbiological data
The Committee considered toxicological data on both compounds, including the results of pharmacokinetic, acute and short-term toxicity, and teratogenicity studies, as well as the results of ototoxicity and clinical studies. The Committee also reviewed an evaluation report on each compound (Annex 1, reference *104*), together with the results of chronic toxicity and *in vitro* microbiological studies on dihydrostreptomycin.

Both streptomycin and dihydrostreptomycin are poorly absorbed following oral administration and most of the dose is recovered unchanged in the faeces in humans and domestic animals.

After parenteral administration of either drug to laboratory or target animals, peak plasma levels are reached within about one hour.

After parenteral administration of aminoglycoside antibiotics to humans, including dihydrostreptomycin and streptomycin, approximately 80% of the dose is recovered in the urine. However, no metabolites have yet been identified. The elimination half-life after therapeutic doses is 2 hours in adults and 5-6 hours in neonates, owing to their lower glomerular filtration rate. Dihydrostreptomycin and streptomycin, in common with other aminoglycoside antibiotics, can be detected in the kidney after depletion from plasma. Residues can be detected in the urine for several weeks after treatment, which suggests that the two drugs accumulate in the kidney.

Accumulation also occurs in the perilymph of the inner ear and both streptomycin and dihydrostreptomycin are known to be ototoxic at therapeutic doses. The risk of ototoxic effects is increased when renal function is compromised.

Placental transfer occurs and fetal serum concentrations range from 20-40% of maternal serum levels.

Single oral doses of dihydrostreptomycin and streptomycin salts were slightly toxic to experimental animals. The median lethal dose (LD_{50}) for dihydrostreptomycin in mice ranged from 12.5 g per kg of body weight for the hydrochloride to over 30 g per kg of body weight for the sulfate. For streptomycin, the LD_{50} in mice ranged from 8.75 g per kg of body weight for the calcium chloride complex to 25 g per kg of body weight for the sulfate.

Parenteral administration of streptomycin at doses of 50-100 mg per kg of body weight per day to dogs for 20 days resulted in renal damage within 1-2 weeks, and three out of five animals developed ataxia.

Ototoxicity was examined in a 90-day study in guinea-pigs treated orally with 40 mg of dihydrostreptomycin per kg of body weight per day. Interpretation of the histopathological data was hampered by inadequate fixation of the cochlea; however, no hearing loss was reported. In a further 90-day study in cats treated orally with 40 mg of dihydro-streptomycin per kg of body weight per day, no treatment-related effects were observed and vestibular function was normal. The no-observed-effect-level (NOEL) in this study was 40 mg per kg of body weight per day.

In a series of studies with streptomycin in monkeys, subcutaneous injection of 25 mg per kg of body weight per day for 66 days caused anaemia. After intravenous administration of 25-50 mg per kg of body weight per day in three divided doses for 5 days, transient impairment of hepatic function was observed. After parenteral administration (by intramuscular, subcutaneous or intravenous injection) of 100-200 mg per kg of body weight per day for 5 days, proteinuria was observed in addition to hepatic impairment. Parenteral doses of 25 mg per kg of body weight per day or more for 5 days caused fatty changes in the liver and to a lesser extent in the kidney. There was no decrease in liver glycogen. These changes were reversible and had disappeared by 66 days after the last injection.

No adverse effects were observed in target animal safety studies in which cattle, sheep and pigs were treated intramuscularly with 30 mg per kg of body weight per day each of dihydrostreptomycin and benzylpenicillin for 5 days (three times the therapeutic dose), or 10 mg per kg of body weight per day of each drug for 15 days (three times the recommended duration of treatment).

Limited information was available on the genotoxicity of dihydro-streptomycin and streptomycin. Streptomycin gave conflicting results in *in vitro* chromosomal aberration tests.

In a 2-year toxicity study in rats, dihydrostreptomycin was administered in the diet to groups of 35 males and 35 females. Drug concentrations were adjusted weekly to give dose levels of 1, 5 or 10 mg per kg of body weight per day. Ten animals from each group (five of each sex) were killed at 6 months and 12 months; the remaining animals were killed at 2 years. After 6 months, a slight (but not dose-related) decrease in body-weight gain was observed in all treated males. At 18 months and 2 years, the body weights of males dosed with 10 mg per kg of body weight per day were slightly lower than those of controls. The incidence of tumours in treated groups at 2 years was no higher than in controls. The survival rate among the treated animals ranged from 12 to 17 out of 25. Although this study did not meet current standards regarding the number of animals used, the Committee concluded that it was adequate for the purpose of evaluating the carcinogenic potential of dihydro-streptomycin. The NOEL was 5 mg per kg of body weight per day, based on the decrease in body-weight gain observed in males at the highest dose.

The Committee concluded that the question of carcinogenic potential of streptomycin had been satisfactorily assessed in the 2-year oral toxicity study with dihydrostreptomycin in rats, since the chemical structure, pharmacokinetic properties and toxicity profile of the two compounds are almost identical.

A number of studies were available in which pregnant mice were treated parenterally with streptomycin at doses of up to 250 mg per kg of body weight per day on various days covering days 9–16 of gestation. Body weights were reduced in both males and females of the F_1 generation at the lowest dose, and vestibular function was impaired at the highest dose. Streptomycin crossed the placental barrier and was identified in the tissue fluids of embryos from treated dams. There was no effect on litter size, and no fetal malformations were observed at any dose.

Daily intramuscular injection of either dihydrostreptomycin or strep-tomycin to pregnant guinea-pigs at doses of 25–200 mg per kg of body weight per day caused abortions or death. No abortions were produced with either drug at a dose of 10 mg per kg of body weight per day. There was evidence of placental damage at this dose level with both compounds, but no teratogenic effects were produced. Vestibular and auditory function were normal in animals of the F_1 generation.

No teratogenic effects were observed in pregnant rabbits treated orally with 5 or 10 mg of dihydrostreptomycin per kg of body weight per day on days 6–18 of gestation. However, no maternal toxicity was observed at these doses, indicating that the dose levels may not have been high enough to exclude teratogenic potential.

The Committee examined a literature review on pregnancy outcomes in 206 women given parenteral streptomycin or dihydrostreptomycin for tuberculosis. The dose administered, where stated, was 1–2 g daily or twice weekly, with total doses ranging from 2 to 202 g. Other drugs were given concomitantly for tuberculosis in 162 cases. The only abnormalities observed were of the inner ear in 35/207 infants (a rate of approximately one in six). These consisted of vestibular dysfunction and varying degrees of hearing loss. Hearing loss occurred in the high-frequency range first, i.e. before the frequencies associated with normal speech were affected.

The Committee considered that the data in animals and humans indicated that the effects of dihydrostreptomycin and streptomycin on the inner ear of fetuses were a manifestation of fetotoxicity. The Committee concluded that these compounds were not teratogenic.

No studies were available on either compound on fertility, perinatal or postnatal effects. Dihydrostreptomycin has been used in veterinary medicine to preserve semen, as well as for the treatment of intrauterine infections and orchitis in humans. In these situations, no adverse effects on reproduction have been reported. However, these data did not adequately address the potential for effects on fertility or reproduction.

Minor renal tubular dysfunction, such as urinary casts and minor degrees of albuminuria, occurs occasionally in humans treated with streptomycin. However, severe renal damage (proximal tubular necrosis) is rare and renal effects are usually reversible on cessation of therapy.

In a study in dogs, dihydrostreptomycin administered in the feed at a dose equivalent to 50 μg per kg of body weight per day caused the development of resistance in the lactose-fermenting coliforms of the intestinal flora. The Committee considered that this study was not appropriate for extrapolation to effects in humans. The dog was considered to be a more sensitive species than humans for these effects because of its shorter intestinal length compared to body mass, and reduced potential for dilution of intestinal contents with other food and intestinal secretions and reduced absorption by intestinal epithelial cells.

Dihydrostreptomycin and streptomycin have a similar spectrum of antimicrobial and biological activity. Accordingly, the Committee used the results of *in vitro* antimicrobial activity studies on dihydro-streptomycin to calculate the upper limit of a hypothetical temporary ADI for combined residues of both compounds as follows:

$$
\text{Upper limit of hypothetical temporary ADI} = \frac{\text{Concentration without effect on human gut flora (µg/ml)} \times \text{Daily faecal bolus (g)}}{\text{Fraction of oral dose bioavailable} \times \text{Safety factor} \times \text{Weight of human (60 kg)}}
$$

$$
= \frac{32 \times 150}{1 \times 1 \times 60}
$$

$$
= 80 \text{ µg per kg of body weight}
$$

It took the following factors into account:

- Factors to account for the range of MICs needed to allow for sensitive bacteria, anaerobic environment, bacterial density and pH: the Committee considered that the MIC values measured at high cell density (10^7 bacteria/well) and under anaerobic conditions were more representative of conditions occurring in the human gut than those measured at lower cell density (10^5 bacteria/well). Data were available on 17 species, including the 10 most common genera of the human gut flora, with 5–11 strains tested per species. The most sensitive species were *Bifidobacterium* spp. An MIC_{50} value for dihydrostreptomycin of 32 µg/ml (equivalent to 32 µg/g) was selected as the concentration without effect on the human gut flora.
- Availability: the Committee noted that no information was available on the binding of drug residues to gut contents. It therefore took a conservative approach, assuming that the availability of orally ingested dihydrostreptomycin and streptomycin to the colonic micro-flora was 100%.
- Variability among exposed individuals: the Committee noted that the colonic flora is relatively stable and that variability between individuals is similar to that within a particular individual. It also noted that other values selected for this calculation were conservative and already incorporated an adequate margin of safety. A safety factor of 1 was therefore selected.

Taking into account the hypothetical temporary ADI based on antimicrobial activity and the available toxicological information, the Committee concluded that the most sensitive effects caused by dihydrostreptomycin and streptomycin were those observed with dihydrostreptomycin in the 2-year oral toxicity study in rats, where the NOEL was 5 mg per kg of body weight per day. Based on this NOEL and using a safety factor of 200, the Committee established a temporary ADI of 0–30 µg per kg of body weight for the combined residues of both dihydrostreptomycin and streptomycin. The ADI was rounded to one significant figure, consistent with accepted rounding procedures (Annex 1, reference *91*, section 2.7).

Residue data

Streptomycin and dihydrostreptomycin are active against a wide range of Gram-negative organisms and some Gram-positive pathogens in cattle, horses, pigs, sheep and humans. There are numerous preparations containing dihydrostreptomycin alone or in combination with either streptomycin or other antibiotics for veterinary use. The combination of penicillin and dihydrostreptomycin is widely used in the treatment of mixed infections involving both Gram-negative and Gram-positive organisms (e.g. mastitis in dairy cattle). The preparations under consideration were administered intramuscularly at a dose of approximately 10 mg of streptomycin/dihydrostreptomycin per kg of body weight per day or injected into the bovine mammary gland over a wide range of doses. The length of treatment depends on the resolution of the infection; however, in the case of preparations containing procaine benzylpenicillin and dihydrostreptomycin, treatment should not exceed 3–5 days.

Dihydrostreptomycin and streptomycin were previously reviewed at the twelfth meeting of the Committee (Annex 1, reference *17*), at which time the recommended MRLs were: meat – 1000 µg/kg; milk – 200 µg/kg; and eggs – 500 µg/kg.

At the present meeting, streptomycin and dihydrostreptomycin were evaluated together because their pharmacokinetic and residue patterns are similar and because their residues are not distinguished from each other by either microbial inhibition assays or enzyme immunoassay methods.

Both drugs were absorbed rapidly from the site of intramuscular injection in cattle, sheep and pigs and were thought to be distributed in the extracellular fluids. They were cleared rapidly from the blood. After intramuscular injection, peak plasma levels were reached within 0.5–1.7 hours, and the half-life was 1.4-4.9 hours. Following parenteral administration of ^{3}H-labelled dihydrostreptomycin, the drug was excreted rapidly in the urine of pigs and cattle. The values of the apparent volume of distribution in both species agreed (21% and 23% of body weight) with estimates for extracellular fluid. These results, together with the lack of activity in both saliva and lacrimal fluids, indicate that dihydrostreptomycin neither equilibrates with intracellular fluids nor accumulates intracellularly. There was a good correlation between the antimicrobial activity and concentration of residues in the blood and urine of pigs and cattle. In the case of intramammary injections containing dihydrostreptomycin, the drug was excreted at varying rates into the milk, depending on the formulations used.

There was very little information on the metabolism of either compound in farm animals, although the drugs are probably not substantially metabolized. No evidence was presented of interconversion of streptomycin and dihydrostreptomycin in tissues of farm animals.

There were no radiodepletion studies reported to determine the total residues in tissues.

Numerous residue studies were presented in which cattle, sheep and pigs were administered a variety of preparations containing unlabelled streptomycin or dihydrostreptomycin intramuscularly at the recommended doses. The residues were measured by either a microbial inhibition assay or an enzyme immunoassay. These methods do not distinguish between the two compounds and cross-reactions may occur with possible metabolites. After intramuscular administration of two preparations containing both dihydrostreptomycin and procaine benzylpenicillin, residue levels in cattle were highest and most persistent in the kidney (see Table 1).

Residue levels in muscle, liver and fat decreased fairly rapidly to below the limit of detection (0.03–1 mg/kg, depending on the tissue and study). There was wide variability in the disappearance of the residues, depending mainly on the formulation of the preparation. Dihydro-streptomycin persisted at the injection site in cattle, sheep and pigs in low amounts (ranging from below 0.8 mg/kg to 5.6 mg/kg) for 3 weeks but was below 0.8 mg/kg in all animals at 4 weeks.

Table 1
Total residues (mg of dihydrostreptomycin per kg) in kidney tissues of cattle, sheep and pigs given two preparations (A and B) containing a combination of dihydrostreptomycin and procaine benzylpenicillin

Withdrawal time (days)	Preparation	Total residues[a]		
		Cattle	Sheep	Pigs
7	A	10.5	15.8	12.6
	B	11–56[b]	4.0–4.2	9–26[b]
14	A	NM	NM	NM
	B	5–19	1.0–1.5	1.4–4.3
18	A	<1	<1	<1
	B	NM	NM	NM
21	A	NM	NM	NM
	B	1.8–2.0	0.05–0.9	1.0–1.9
28	A	NM	NM	NM
	B	<0.4–0.5	<0.8	<0.4

NM: not measured.
[a] Values were measured by a microbial inhibition assay for preparation A and by an enzyme immunoassay for preparation B.
[b] Samples were collected on day 6.

Residues of dihydrostreptomycin and streptomycin in the milk of cattle treated with a variety of intramuscular and intramammary preparations containing dihydrostreptomycin were measured by an enzyme immunoassay, a receptor-binding assay or microbial inhibition assays. The residue levels decreased below the MRL recommended at the twelfth meeting of the Committee (200 μg/kg; Annex 1, reference *17*) between 3 and 15 milkings after drug administration, depending on the formulation of the preparation. The Committee recommended that kidney, muscle and milk should serve as target tissues for dihydrostreptomycin and streptomycin residues.

A residue-depletion study was reported, in which laying hens were administered a single intramuscular injection of 100 mg of dihydrostreptomycin per kg of body weight. Residue levels were above 500 μg/kg in whole egg for at least 8 days after drug administration. Laying hens were also administered the drug in the drinking-water at a level of 1 g/l (equivalent to 100 mg per kg of body weight) for 5 consecutive days. Residue levels in eggs were below the limits of detection (300 μg/kg for albumin, 3000 μg/kg for yolk), which suggested that dihydrostreptomycin was poorly absorbed from the gastrointestinal tract.

No data were presented on the bioavailability of bound residues.

Methods of analysis
The analytical microbial inhibition assays and enzyme immunoassay methods for measuring residues of streptomycin and dihydrostreptomycin are adequate for screening purposes, with detection limits well below 1 mg/kg for tissues. In milk the enzyme immunoassay methods have claimed limits of detection of 5–20 μg/l, whereas in the microbial inhibition assays the limits of detection are 100–200 μg/l. Although many data were available, neither method was fully validated nor was the enzyme immunoassay performed according to Good Laboratory Practice standards. The Committee noted that the quantification limits of the HPLC and thin-layer chromatography (TLC) methods reported in the literature for measuring aminoglycoside residues in animal tissues were 20 μg/kg for streptomycin and 40 μg/kg for dihydrostreptomycin in muscle and kidney and 10 μg/kg and 20 μg/kg respectively in milk. An analytical method based on liquid chromatography and mass spectrometry was reported for measuring residues in bovine kidney with limits of quantification of 440 μg/kg and 320 μg/kg for streptomycin and dihydrostreptomycin, respectively.

Maximum Residue Limits
Based on the temporary ADI of 0–30 μg/kg for streptomycin and dihydrostreptomycin established by the Committee, the permitted daily intake of the parent drugs and/or their equivalents is 1800 μg for a 60-kg person.

The following factors were taken into account in estimating the MRLs:

- The temporary ADI, which was based on a toxicological end-point.
- The limits of detection or quantification of the analytical methods.
- The marker residue for edible tissues and milk is the sum of the streptomycin and dihydrostreptomycin residues.
- The ratio of the marker residues to the total residues is uncertain, although it was predicted that there is little metabolism of either drug and the ratio may be close to unity.

The Committee recommended temporary MRLs of 500 µg/kg for muscle, liver and fat and 1000 µg/kg for kidney in cattle, sheep, pigs and chickens, and 200 µg/l for milk in cattle, expressed as the sum of the concentrations of streptomycin and dihydrostreptomycin. If the recommended values are used for the MRLs and account is taken of the factors mentioned above, the theoretical maximum intake of residue of streptomycin and dihydrostreptomycin, based on ingestion of 300 g of muscle, 100 g of liver, 50 g each of kidney and fat and 1.5 l of milk, is 575 µg per day.

Insufficient data were available to maintain the MRL of 500 µg/kg for residues in eggs set at the twelfth meeting of the Committee.

The following information is required for evaluation in 1997:

1. Information to assess the potential for effects on fertility and perinatal and postnatal toxicity.
2. An evaluation report or results of experimental studies on the metabolism of dihydrostreptomycin and streptomycin.
3. Data on residues of streptomycin and dihydrostreptomycin in eggs.
4. Results of studies to determine the relationship between the antimicrobial activity of the residues and their concentration, as measured by specific chemical methods.

3.2.2 *Enrofloxacin*

Enrofloxacin had not been previously evaluated by the Committee. It is a quinolone antimicrobial that is most effective against Gram-negative bacteria and is used for treating respiratory, gastrointestinal and urinary tract infections in cattle, pigs and poultry. Enrofloxacin acts via the inhibition of DNA gyrase (EC 5.99.1.3).

Toxicological and microbiological data
The Committee considered toxicological data on enrofloxacin, including the results of acute, short-term and long-term toxicity studies and studies on carcinogenicity, reproductive and developmental toxicity, mutagenicity, metabolism and residues. It also considered information on antimicrobial effects and observations in humans following treatment with ciprofloxacin, the major metabolite of enrofloxacin.

In rats orally dosed with 5 mg per kg of body weight of radiolabelled enrofloxacin, 75% of the dose was absorbed. Enrofloxacin was rapidly absorbed and distributed to all tissues, with the highest levels in the liver and kidneys. Enrofloxacin was rapidly excreted via the urine and bile. The urine contained mainly unchanged parent drug and the de-ethylated compound, ciprofloxacin. Approximately 40% of the dose was excreted in the bile, primarily as unchanged enrofloxacin. Similar results were obtained with all species of animals tested.

Enrofloxacin is a relatively stable molecule. It is primarily metabolized in the liver, with the main metabolite in all species being ciprofloxacin, probably formed by oxidative dealkylation. In rats four other metabolites were identified, each accounting for less than 2% of the total residue.

Single oral or topical doses of enrofloxacin were slightly toxic to experimental animals (LD_{50} = 500–5000 mg per kg of body weight). In mice, single intravenous doses were moderately toxic (LD_{50} = 220 mg per kg of body weight).

In a 90-day study in rats in which enrofloxacin was administered in the feed, chronic degenerative changes in the auricular cartilage were seen at doses equal to 150 and 577 mg per kg of body weight per day. Treatment-related morphological changes in the spermatozoa and atrophy of the testicular tubules were observed in males at 577 mg per kg of body weight per day. These effects were not observed in the group treated at a dose equal to 36 mg per kg of body weight per day.

A special study was performed to assess further the morphological changes in the reproductive tract observed in male rats in previous studies. Male rats were administered enrofloxacin in the feed at dose levels equal to 10, 38 or 615 mg per kg of body weight per day for 90 days, followed by a 90-day recovery period. Statistically significant decreases in epididymal weights were seen at 91 days in the groups given 38 and 615 mg per kg of body weight per day. The testes/body weight and epididymides/body weight ratios were significantly lower than in controls at 615 mg per kg of body weight per day. In addition, two of 30 rats showed bilateral testicular atrophy after the 90-day recovery period. Abnormal spermatozoa were observed at 615 mg per kg of body weight per day at days 14 and 91 but not at the end of the 90-day recovery period. The NOEL for testicular toxicity in this study was 10 mg per kg of body weight per day.

To assess effects on testicular toxicity and articular cartilage in young dogs, a 90-day study in 3-4-month-old dogs was performed in which enrofloxacin was administered orally at dose levels equal to 3, 9.6 or 75 mg per kg of body weight per day. All treated animals except those given the lowest dose showed degeneration of the articular cartilage. The testes/body weight ratio for treated animals was consistently higher than for controls, although this was not statistically significant. In addition, in all four male dogs in the highest-dose group and one of four in the lowest-dose group, marked dilatation of the seminiferous tubules and focal areas of single-layer spermatogonial cells or vacuolated epithelium in the tubules were considered beyond normal limits. It could not be determined whether the testicular changes observed in the lowest-dose group were treatment-related or due to the fact that the animals were not fully mature. Therefore, the Committee was not able to derive a NOEL for this study. The Committee noted that no such effects were observed in 12–13-month-old dogs dosed orally with enrofloxacin at up to 52 mg per kg of body weight per day for 90 days.

A 90-day study was performed in 3-month-old male dogs dosed orally with enrofloxacin at levels equal to 0.3, 0.6, 1.2 or 92 mg per kg of body weight per day to investigate further the testicular effects of enrofloxacin observed in the earlier study with 3–4-month-old dogs. At the termination of the study, testicular weights were determined and testes and epididymides collected for histopathological assessment. No other tissues were examined. Testicular weights and testes/body weight ratios were higher than those of controls at 0.3, 0.6 and 1.2 mg per kg of body weight per day. In addition, lameness was seen in the highest-dose group after 2–3 days of treatment. This effect was not seen at 1.2 mg per kg of body weight per day. One of four dogs in the highest-dose group also had bilateral testicular degenerative changes. The NOEL for lameness in this study was 1.2 mg per kg of body weight per day.

A 90-day study with a 90-day recovery period was conducted, in which 3-month-old male dogs were dosed orally with enrofloxacin at levels equal to 0.3 or 1.2 mg per kg of body weight per day to investigate the possibility of testicular effects being delayed until after the animals reached sexual maturity. After the recovery period, gross and microscopic examination of testes and epididymides showed no evidence of toxicity. Testes and epididymides from all treated animals appeared mature and contained normal, mature spermatozoa. There was no evidence of delayed testicular toxicity at either dose level. The NOEL in this study was 1.2 mg per kg of body weight per day.

Enrofloxacin was not carcinogenic in mice dosed orally at levels equal to 323, 1100 or 3520 mg per kg of body weight per day in a 2-year toxicity/carcinogenicity study. Intrahepatic and extrahepatic bile duct hyperplasia was seen in males in the mid-dose group and in both sexes in the highest-dose group. The NOEL was 323 mg per kg of body weight per day.

On the basis of a long-term toxicity/carcinogenicity study in which rats were dosed orally at levels equal to 41, 103, 338 or 856 mg per kg of body weight per day, the Committee concluded that enrofloxacin was not carcinogenic in this species. However, a NOEL could not be determined for the bile duct hyperplasia observed in this study. The NOEL for bile duct hyperplasia in further limited long-term studies with enrofloxacin in rats was 2.9 mg per kg of body weight per day.

A two-generation reproductive toxicity study in rats was performed with enrofloxacin administered in the feed at doses up to a level equal to 630 mg per kg of body weight per day. An increase in the length of gestation, and reductions in the number of litters, litter size and number of implants in the parental and first filial generations were observed in the highest-dose group. Survival and growth rates were significantly decreased in the progeny of these animals. Alterations in the morphology of the spermatozoa were noted in males in the highest-dose group in both the parental and first filial generations and were considered the primary cause for the adverse effects on fertility. The NOEL for reproductive effects in this study was 165 mg per kg of body weight per day.

An additional two-generation reproductive study was performed in rats in which enrofloxacin was administered in the feed at doses equivalent to 6.25, 15 or 100 mg per kg of body weight per day. The purpose of the study was to determine whether the drug affected gonadal function and mating behaviour in treated males or reproductive parameters in females, and to monitor growth and development of the offspring of the parental and first filial generation. Administration of enrofloxacin caused a reduction in mean epididymal weights at the highest dose and alterations in sperm morphology at 15 and 100 mg per kg of body weight per day. No effects on fertility or reproductive performance were noted. The NOEL was 6.25 mg per kg of body weight per day.

A special fertility study was performed in sexually mature male rats, in which enrofloxacin was given in the diet at a dose equivalent to 375 mg per kg of body weight per day for 90 days. The purpose of the study was to determine the timing of the onset of spermatic dysmorphogenesis and to ascertain whether functional fertility was restored during a 90-day recovery phase. Administration of enrofloxacin caused a significant decrease in male fertility, food consumption and body-weight gain. Testes weights were increased during treatment, but were lower than in controls at the end of the recovery period. Treatment-related dys-morphogenic changes in the spermatozoa were seen by week 3 and these changes were partially reversible, since functional fertility returned to 13 of 15 previously treated males. Six of these animals demonstrated varying degrees of atrophy of the seminiferous tubules and other degenerative alterations.

In a teratology study in rats, enrofloxacin was administered by gavage at doses of 50, 210 or 875 mg per kg of body weight per day on days 6–15 of gestation. Maternal toxicity was observed at 210 and 875 mg per kg of body weight per day. Although food consumption was higher than in controls in the highest-dose group, mean maternal weight gain was significantly lower in these animals. Fetal weights and litter size were significantly lower and the number of fetal resorptions and post-implantation losses was higher in the highest-dose group. Fetal weights were also significantly lower in the mid-dose group. Skeletal examination of fetuses in the mid- and highest-dose groups revealed delayed skeletal ossification, which correlated with the decreased fetal weights. No teratogenic effects were observed. The NOEL in this study was 50 mg per kg of body weight per day.

In *in vitro* genotoxicity tests, enrofloxacin gave equivocal results in a forward-mutation test in mammalian cells and positive results in chromosomal aberration tests. Negative results were obtained in *in vivo* genotoxicity tests, including bone marrow micronucleus, sister chromatid exchange and bone marrow chromosomal aberration tests. The Committee concluded that enrofloxacin is not genotoxic.

The potential for adverse effects on the human gastrointestinal flora was considered from summary data. The results of *in vitro* MIC investigations using ciprofloxacin and strains representative of the human gut flora were submitted for assessment. *Escherichia coli* was found to be the most sensitive bacterium, with an MIC_{50} value of 0.015 µg/ml (equivalent to 0.015 µg/g).

In calculating the ADI, the Committee used the formula developed at the thirty-eighth meeting of the Committee (Annex 1, reference 97):

$$\text{Upper limit of temporary ADI} = \frac{\text{Concentration without effect on human gut flora (µg/ml)} \times \text{Daily faecal bolus (g)}}{\text{Fraction of oral dose bioavailable} \times \text{Safety factor} \times \text{Weight of human (60 kg)}}$$

$$= \frac{(0.015 \times 20) \times 150}{0.12 \times 10 \times 60}$$

$$\approx 0.6 \text{ µg per kg of body weight}$$

It took the following factors into account:

- Factors to account for the range of MICs needed to allow for sensitive bacteria, anaerobic environment, bacterial density and pH: since the MIC for *E. coli* was determined using an inoculum density of 10^5 bacteria/ml, a factor of 20 was used to account for the higher density of bacteria in the human intestine. For example, MIC values for Enterobacteriaceae and *Pseudomonas aeruginosa* increased 8–32-fold when the inoculum density was increased to 10^7 bacteria/ml.
- Availability: the fraction of the dose available to the gut microflora was derived from studies of ciprofloxacin in humans. In human volunteers who had received two oral doses of 50 mg of ciprofloxacin, the faecal concentration was found to be 80 mg/kg. In 150 g of faeces, this corresponds to 12% of the orally ingested dose.
- Variability among exposed individuals: an additional safety factor of 10 was used to account for the possible variation in absorption between ciprofloxacin and enrofloxacin, uncertainty relating to the biliary excretion of enrofloxacin, and variability between individuals.

In view of the absence of information on the effects on enrofloxacin on microorganisms obtained from the human intestine, a temporary ADI of 0–0.6 μg per kg of body weight was established, based on the results of the limited summary data on microbiological tests on ciprofloxacin. The Committee noted that the temporary ADI provided an adequate margin of safety in relation to the NOEL of 1.2 mg per kg of body weight per day for testicular toxicity in dogs.

Residue data

Enrofloxacin has a wide spectrum of antimicrobial activity. It is administered either orally or parenterally to cattle and pigs at doses of 2.5–5 mg per kg of body weight and orally to poultry at 10–12 mg per kg of body weight. There is some use in lactating dairy cows and laying hens. The normal treatment period is 3–5 days.

Enrofloxacin is rapidly absorbed from the gut in cattle and poultry, with plasma concentrations reaching peak values within 8 hours. The route of excretion in farm animals has not been investigated.

The metabolism of enrofloxacin was studied in farm animals and rats, using the ^{14}C-labelled compound. The main residues were parent drug and ciprofloxacin except in poultry muscle and skin, where only parent drug was present. This is in contrast to bovine tissue, where ciprofloxacin was the most abundant residue.

The depletion of the total residues of [2-^{14}C]enrofloxacin was measured in calves, pigs, chickens and turkeys. There were large standard deviations of the means for the residue concentration values for most tissues. The rate of depletion was not constant during the elimination phase. However, except in the case of bovine liver, the residue concentrations were below 500 μg/kg in all edible tissues by the third day after the last drug administration. The residues were most persistent in poultry skin and bovine liver and kidney tissues.

Residues of enrofloxacin and ciprofloxacin were measured by an HPLC method in the edible tissues, milk and eggs of farm animals following oral or parenteral administration of multiple doses of enrofloxacin, as recommended by the sponsors. Residues were also measured at the injection site following parenteral administration. In calves, the concentrations of ciprofloxacin and enrofloxacin residues were below 100 μg/kg in all tissues at 3 days after dosing. Enrofloxacin was administered by intravenous injection to lactating dairy cows for 5 consecutive days at a dose of 2.5 mg per kg of body weight in one study and 5 mg per kg of body weight in a second study. The concentration of both residues in the milk decreased rapidly and enrofloxacin was not detectable after day 2, whereas ciprofloxacin was not detectable (limit of detection 2 μg/kg) in samples collected from day 5 onwards. Pigs received enrofloxacin orally at a dose of 2.5 mg per kg of body weight for 3 consecutive days. The concentrations of residues of enrofloxacin and ciprofloxacin were low (the highest levels were 290 µg/kg and 100 µg/kg respectively in kidney) 1 day after dosing and decreased rapidly, so that at day 3 withdrawal ciprofloxacin was not detected and enrofloxacin was found only in the liver and kidney tissues. No residues were detected at 7 or 14 days withdrawal nor were any residues detected following administration of enrofloxacin in the feed. In chickens given enrofloxacin in the drinking-water at a dose of 41 mg/l, residues in the liver depleted rapidly to about 200 µg/kg over a 3-day period after treatment. In broilers administered enrofloxacin in their drinking-water at a dose of 25 mg/l, the concentration of residues was about 20 µg/kg in skin at 2 days after dosing and below the limit of detection (10 µg/kg) in eggs at 10 days after dosing. When the recommended dose of 50 mg/l of drinking-water was administered, the residues were higher and persisted for a longer period. For example, enrofloxacin and ciprofloxacin residue levels in skin were 120 µg/kg and 20 µg/kg respectively at day 4, 100 µg/kg and 20 µg/kg at day 7, and 50 µg/kg and below the limit of detection at day 10. Residues of enrofloxacin but not ciprofloxacin were detected in liver tissue of broilers for at least 17 days after dosing.

Methods of analysis

The analytical methods used by the sponsor are based on homogenization of tissue and extraction of both enrofloxacin and ciprofloxacin into an organic phase. The extract may be further purified and dissolved in the HPLC mobile phase. After resolution by HPLC, the residue levels are measured by either ultraviolet or fluorescence detection. Recently these methods have been improved by using a mobile phase containing tetrabutylammonium bisulfate in water and acetonitrile and changing the HPLC conditions. These methods have a claimed limit of detection of 1 µg/kg and a limit of quantification of 10 µg/kg for most tissues.

Maximum Residue Limits

Based on the temporary ADI of 0–0.6 µg/kg for enrofloxacin established by the Committee, the permitted daily intake of parent drug and/or its equivalents is 36 µg for a 60-kg person.

In reaching its decision on MRLs, the Committee considered the following factors:

- The temporary ADI was based on a microbiological end-point.
- The quantification limits of the analytical methods (10 µg/kg for enrofloxacin and ciprofloxacin in tissues and 5 µg/kg in milk).
- The marker residue for tissues is the sum of the enrofloxacin and ciprofloxacin residues. Ciprofloxacin is the marker residue for bovine milk.
- Neither the ratio of marker residues to total residues nor the percentage of total residues associated with antimicrobial activity was known.

Since enrofloxacin and ciprofloxacin account for only 20% of total residues in pig liver, the intake of antimicrobially active residues could be up to five times the concentration of the marker residues.

The Committee noted that even if the MRLs were based on the limits of quantification of the most sensitive analytical methods multiplied by a factor of 2, the intake of marker residues from muscle, liver, kidney, fat, milk and eggs would be 39 µg (Table 2), which is close to the maximum ADI of 36 µg.

However, the Committee noted that the hypothetical MRLs based on the limits of quantification of the analytical method would not take into account any antimicrobial activity of the significant fraction (up to 80%) forming the remaining residues. It therefore concluded that it was not possible to allocate MRLs to enrofloxacin.

The following information is required for evaluation in 1997:

1. Detailed reports of the *in vitro* MIC investigations of enrofloxacin that were submitted for evaluation.
2. Information on the effects of enrofloxacin and ciprofloxacin on specific genera of microorganisms obtained from the human intestine.

In addition, the Committee required that the results of studies to determine the antimicrobial activity of the residues other than enrofloxacin and ciprofloxacin be submitted for review as soon as they become available.

Table 2
Minimum residue levels of enrofloxacin that could be considered as a basis for MRL calculations[a]

Tissue	Theoretical MRL (µg/kg)[b]	Theoretical maximum daily intake (µg)
Muscle	40	12
Liver	40	4
Kidney	40	2
Fat	40	2
Milk	10	15
Eggs	40	4

[a] Based on a daily intake of 0.5 kg of meat made up of 0.3 kg of muscle, 0.1 kg of liver, 0.05 kg of kidney and 0.05 kg of fat, 1.5 kg of milk, and 0.1 kg of egg.
[b] Based on the limit of quantification for the sum of enrofloxacin and ciprofloxacin residues in tissues and for ciprofloxacin residues in milk, multiplied by a factor of 2.

3.2.3 *Gentamicin*

Gentamicin had not previously been reviewed by the Committee. It is an aminoglycoside antibiotic that is effective against a wide variety of microorganisms.

Toxicological and microbiological data

The toxicological data considered by the Committee included the results of studies on pharmacokinetics and metabolism, of acute and short-term toxicity studies, and of studies on reproductive toxicity, teratogenicity, genotoxicity and antimicrobial activity. The Committee also considered information from a variety of special studies and observations in humans.

Gentamicin, in common with other aminoglycoside drugs, is poorly absorbed from the gastrointestinal tract. Parenteral doses are mainly distributed into the extracellular fluid, although there is significant penetration into the cortex of the kidney and the inner ear. There is negligible metabolism of the drug and unchanged gentamicin is excreted rapidly, mostly in the urine.

Single oral doses of gentamicin were slightly toxic in rodents (LD_{50} = 8000–10 000 mg per kg of body weight), which supports the view that the drug is largely unabsorbed when administered by this route. In contrast, gentamicin was highly toxic in mice, rats, guinea-pigs and dogs when given intravenously (LD_{50} = 37–67 mg per kg of body weight) and moderately toxic when administered by the intramuscular, subcutaneous and intraperitoneal routes (LD_{50} = 213–893 mg per kg of body weight).

A number of studies was available in which gentamicin was administered by the intramuscular and subcutaneous routes to rats at doses of up to 200 mg per kg of body weight per day and dogs at doses of up to 100 mg per kg of body weight per day for periods of up to 12 months and to monkeys at doses of up to 75 mg per kg of body weight per day for 3 weeks. The kidney was the primary target organ in each species, with effects being observed predominantly in the renal cortex. The major findings were an increase in interstitial nephritis and toxic nephrosis in the proximal convoluted tubules. The latter was characterized by a dose- and time-dependent progression from loss of brush borders of the epithelium, to cloudy swelling of the tubules, the presence of casts and proteinaceous material, desquamation of epithelial cells and necrosis. These changes were associated with a profound impairment of renal function and, in extreme cases, death of severely affected animals. Special studies in rats suggested that the nephrotoxicity may be associated with disruption of lysosomal function. Nephrotoxicity has been observed in humans treated with gentamicin.

Toxic effects on the inner ear have been reported following exposure to aminoglycosides, including gentamicin. There were no clear indications of ototoxicity in the general toxicity studies; however, in a special study in monkeys, gentamicin administered at doses of up to 50 mg per kg of body weight per day caused a reduction in the number of hair cells and the thickness of sensory epithelium in structures of the ear, as well as a functional loss in hearing. Observations in humans have revealed auditory or vestibular toxicity after therapeutic administration of gentamicin.

In 3-month studies in rats and dogs, gentamicin administered orally at doses of up to 116 and 60 mg per kg of body weight per day, respectively, caused virtually no systemic effects. Soft stools or diarrhoea were observed in both species, and dogs in the highest-dose group showed interstitial nephritis. The NOELs were 19 mg per kg of body weight per day in rats and 10 mg per kg of body weight per day in dogs.

A multigeneration reproductive toxicity study in rats showed no adverse effects on reproductive parameters after intramuscular injections of 5 or 20 mg of gentamicin per kg of body weight per day. Teratogenicity studies in mice, rats, guinea-pigs and rabbits did not identify any potential for the production of fetal abnormalities. However, fetotoxic effects, in the form of fetal deaths in mice (10 mg per kg of body weight per day) and rats (50 mg per kg of body weight per day) and reduced birth weight in rats (75 mg per kg of body weight per day), were observed after parenteral dosing.

Positive results were obtained in some *in vitro* genotoxicity studies, but none of these was considered adequate to evaluate the genotoxicity of gentamicin. There were no carcinogenicity studies available on gentamicin. Toxicity studies of up to one year's duration in experimental animals revealed no preneoplastic or neoplastic lesions. The Committee considered the data to be inadequate to assess fully the carcinogenic potential of gentamicin.

Data on the effect of gentamicin on human gut flora were not available. However, *in vitro* data were presented on MICs for over 600 clinical isolates of anaerobic bacteria, including some species representative of the microbial flora in the human gastrointestinal tract. Many of the organisms were found to be resistant to gentamicin; *Eubacterium* spp. were the most sensitive, with MIC values in the range of 0.1–25 µg/ml (MIC_{50} = 0.8 µg/ml, equivalent to 0.8 µg/g) at an inoculum density of 10^3–10^4 colony-forming units/plate.

In view of the poor absorption of gentamicin from the gastrointestinal tract and the reported occurrence of diarrhoea in experimental animals, the Committee considered that the most likely limiting factor to the consumption of residues would be effects on human gut microflora. In calculating the ADI, the Committee used the formula developed at its thirty-eighth meeting (Annex 1, reference 97):

$$\text{Upper limit of temporary ADI} = \frac{\text{Concentration without effect on human gut flora (µg/ml)} \times \text{Daily faecal bolus (g)}}{\text{Fraction of oral dose bioavailable} \times \text{Safety factor} \times \text{Weight of human (60 kg)}}$$

$$= \frac{(0.8 \times 2) \times 150}{1 \times 1 \times 60}$$

$$= 4 \text{ µg per kg of body weight}$$

The Committee took the following factors into account:

- Factors to account for the range of MICs needed to allow for sensitive bacteria, anaerobic environment, bacterial density and pH: the Committee concluded that a factor of 2 was required to account for the relatively low inoculum density used in the *in vitro* studies.
- Availability: the Committee noted that absorption of gentamicin after oral dosing is very poor. It therefore took a conservative approach, assuming that the availability of ingested gentamicin to bacteria in the gastrointestinal tract was 100%.
- Variability among exposed individuals: MIC data on more than 600 clinical isolates of anaerobic bacteria were available. The Committee noted that the colonic flora is relatively stable and that variability among individuals is similar to that within a particular individual. In addition, it recognized that other values selected for this calculation were conservative and already incorporated an adequate margin of safety. A safety factor of 1 was therefore adopted.

In view of the absence of information on the effects of gentamicin on microorganisms obtained from the human intestine and the need for further genotoxicity studies, the Committee established a temporary ADI of 0–4 µg per kg of body weight based on the results of microbiological testing of clinical isolates, with a request for further information. An additional safety factor was not used to account for the temporary status of the ADI because conservative factors were used in deriving the temporary ADI. The Committee noted that the lowest NOEL based on toxicological studies was 10 mg per kg of body weight per day, which is more than 2000 times the temporary ADI based on a microbiological end-point.

Residue data

Gentamicin, an aminoglycoside antibiotic produced by fermentation of *Micromonospora purpurea*, is a mixture of basic, water-soluble compounds containing the aminocyclitol 2-deoxystreptamine and two additional amino sugars. The three major components are designated C_1, C_2 and C_{1a}, but minor components which may be present in formulations include A, B, B_1 and X. Gentamicin is normally formulated as the sulfate salt and is used for the treatment of a variety of bacterial infections in pigs, poultry, cattle and horses. Various formulations of gentamicin have been produced for use in food-producing animals. Some of these are in combination with other antibiotics, including benzylpenicillin, ampicillin and cloxacillin.

Pharmacokinetic studies in beagle dogs, 1-day-old chicks and 3-month-old pigs were available. Radiometric studies in dogs showed that residue levels were approximately 400 times higher in the kidney cortex than in skeletal muscle. In 1-day-old chicks treated by subcutaneous injection, gentamicin reached peak levels in blood within 30 minutes and was rapidly excreted, with levels in blood declining to 50% 2 hours after dosing. The drug was rapidly distributed throughout the tissues, reaching peak levels in the kidneys 24 hours after treatment. There were insufficient details to evaluate the pharmacokinetic data in pigs.

Residue levels in the kidneys of 6-week-old pigs were determined by total radioactivity, radioimmunoassay and antimicrobial assay following intramuscular or oral administration of [^{3}H]gentamicin. All the assays produced similar results, suggesting no significant loss of antimicrobial activity. Residues of gentamicin were also determined by total radio-activity in the tissues of 3-day-old piglets following a single intra-muscular injection of 5 mg of gentamicin (see Table 3). However, in the 6-week-old piglets, which received the oral dose via their drinking-water, residues were more persistent in the liver than in the kidneys. A further study, in which 3-day-old piglets were given a single oral dose estimated at 3.6 mg of [^{3}H]gentamicin per kg of body weight, demonstrated that residues persisted for up to 11 days in the kidneys and 6 days in the liver, but showed little distribution into muscle tissue.

Three studies were conducted in 3-day-old piglets, which were given a single oral dose of 5 mg of unlabelled gentamicin. Similar residue levels of gentamicin in the kidneys were found at all sampling dates in healthy animals and animals with colibacillosis in the first and second studies, indicating that the health status of the piglets had no significant effect on residue depletion. In the third study, where kidney, liver, muscle and fat samples were collected from healthy animals and analysed 1, 3, 6, 9, 11 and 14 days after treatment, only one liver sample (collected at day 3) contained detectable residues. Residues in kidney samples were below the detection limit of 0.08 mg/kg at day 14. No muscle or fat samples contained detectable residues.

Two studies on administration of gentamicin to calves were available, one of which was complicated by the death of experimental animals during the study. Data were considered for the surviving 19 calves in this study (see Table 4). In the second study, in which animals received gentamicin by combined intramuscular injection and oral administration (4 mg per kg of body weight by each route, followed after 12 hours by an additional 4 mg per kg of body weight orally), residues were shown to persist in kidney from one calf at a concentration of 0.47 mg/kg at 100 days after treatment.

Table 3
Total residues (mg of gentamicin per kg) in tissues of 3-day-old piglets given a single intramuscular dose of [³H]gentamicin at 5 mg[a]

Withdrawal time (days)	Total residues[b]			
	Kidney	Liver	Muscle	Fat
14	0.68	0.42	<0.02 0.12[c]	<0.02
28	0.18	0.11	<0.02 <0.02[c]	<0.02
35	0.07	0.06	<0.02 <0.02[c]	<0.02
42	0.05	0.04	<0.02 <0.02[c]	<0.02
49	0.02	0.02	<0.02 <0.02[c]	<0.02

[a] For tissues at 14 days and 49 days withdrawal time, values are means for two animals and one animal respectively; all other values are means for three animals.
[b] Based on five replicate assays per tissue sample.
[c] Injection site.

Table 4
Residues (mg of gentamicin per kg) in tissues of calves given a single combined oral and intramuscular dose of gentamicin,[a] as determined by cylinder plate assay

Withdrawal time (days)	Total residues[b]		
	Kidney	Liver	Muscle
7	>10	3.6	0.7 NM[c]
30	2.0	0.8	BD BD[c]
60	1.1	0.6	BD BD[c]
70	0.9	0.3	BD NM[c]
80	0.6	0.3	BD NM[c]

BD: below the limit of detection (0.05 mg/kg); NM: not measured.
[a] 4 mg per kg of body weight by each route, followed after 12 hours by an additional 4 mg per kg of body weight orally.
[b] For tissues at 7 and 60 days withdrawal time, values are means for five animals; all other values are means for three animals.
[c] Injection site.

Ten residue-depletion studies were performed in dairy cattle, given gentamicin by intramuscular injection (one study), intramammary infusion (three studies) or intrauterine infusion (six studies). Milk was free of detectable residues at 60–84 hours following intramuscular or intramammary treatment, while no detectable gentamicin residues were found in milk collected at the first milking (6–12 hours) following intrauterine administration. Residues of gentamicin were detected in the kidneys at 30 days after intramammary and intrauterine treatment. Table 5 shows the residue levels found in milk collected from dairy cows receiving gentamicin by intramammary infusion after each of three successive milkings.

Residue-depletion studies in 1-day-old chicks treated with 0.2 mg of gentamicin by subcutaneous injection showed tissue concentrations of residues of gentamicin after 7 days withdrawal, of 0.10 mg/kg in skin and fat, 1.1 mg/kg in liver and 3.3 mg/kg in kidney (limit of detection 0.08 mg/kg). Residues in muscle were below the limit of detection (0.16 mg/kg) at day 7.

With respect to analytical methods, the Committee reviewed details of a radioimmunoassay and a cylinder plate assay. The cylinder plate assay, which uses *Staphylococcus epidermidis* ATCC 12228 as the test organism, had a claimed limit of detection of 0.01 mg/l for gentamicin residues in milk and 0.04–0.16 mg/kg in tissues. A number of

Table 5
Residues (mg of gentamicin per litre) in milk collected from five normal lactating cows given an intramammary infusion of 50 mg of gentamicin sulfate and 100 000 IU of procaine benzylpenicillin into each quarter at each of three successive milkings

Withdrawal time (hours)	Residues				
	Cow 1	Cow 2	Cow 3	Cow 4	Cow 5
12	2.30	2.63	1.21	2.84	1.63
24	0.25	0.25	0.26	0.61	0.16
36	BD[a]	0.06	BD[a]	0.10	BD[a]
48	BD[b]	BD[a]	BD[b]	BD[a]	BD[a]
60	BD[b]	BD[b]	BD[b]	BD[b]	BD[a]
72	BD[b]	BD[b]	BD[b]	BD[b]	BD[b]

BD: below the limit of detection (0.05 mg/l).
[a] Residue levels were below the limit of detection in pooled samples from all four quarters.
[b] Residue levels were below the limit of detection in each individual sample.

commercially available test kits are claimed to be suitable for screening milk and tissue samples for gentamicin residues at concentrations below 1 mg/l and 1 mg/kg, respectively. While no multi-laboratory validations have been reported, a liquid chromatography method has recently been described that meets the performance criteria of the Codex Committee on Residues of Veterinary Drugs in Foods. A recently developed method based on liquid chromatography and mass spectrometry should be suitable for confirming the presence of gentamicin residues in tissues, but the equipment is not currently available in all regulatory laboratories.

Maximum Residue Limits

Based on the temporary ADI of 0–4 µg per kg of body weight established by the Committee using a microbiological end-point, the permitted daily intake of gentamicin would be 240 µg of antimicrobially active gentamicin residues contributed by 500 g of food-animal tissues together with 1.5 l of milk in the diet of a 60-kg person. This is expressed as parent drug, as there was no indication of significant metabolism.

The Committee recommended temporary MRLs for gentamicin of 100 µg/kg for muscle and fat, 200 µg/kg for liver, and 1000 µg/kg for kidney in both cattle and pigs, as well as 100 µg/l for cows' milk, expressed as parent drug.

The temporary MRL allocated to milk takes into account the limit of quantification of current analytical methods. No MRLs were assigned to poultry or eggs because appropriate data were not available. The temporary MRLs recommended above would result in a daily maximum intake of 255 µg of gentamicin residues based on a daily food intake of 300 g of muscle, 100 g of liver, 50 g each of kidney and fat, and 1.5 l of milk (Annex 1, reference *85*).

The following information is required for evaluation in 1997:

1. Results of studies on the effects of gentamicin on specific genera of microorganisms obtained from the human intestine.
2. Additional data to assist in the assessment of carcinogenic potential, which should include:

   (a) results of genotoxicity assays for gene mutations in mammalian cells and chromosomal aberrations *in vitro* and *in vivo*; and
   (b) details of an investigation on possible structural similarities between gentamicin and known carcinogens.

3. A validated chemical analytical method with a limit of quantification below the MRL recommended for milk.

3.2.4 *Neomycin*

The aminoglycosides as a group were evaluated at the twelfth meeting of the Committee (Annex 1, reference *17*). At that time, no ADI was established because of a lack of adequate toxicological and residue data and the Committee recommended that if aminoglycosides were used they should not be allowed to give rise to detectable residue levels in human food. Since then, data specific for neomycin have become available.

Toxicological and microbiological data
The Committee considered toxicological data on neomycin, including the results of acute, short-term, and long-term toxicity studies, as well as studies on pharmacokinetics, reproductive and developmental toxicity, genotoxicity, carcinogenicity, effects in humans and antimicrobial activity. An evaluation report, as requested for veterinary drugs with a long history of use (Annex 1, reference *104*), was also provided.

Neomycin is poorly absorbed after oral administration, whereas after parenteral administration it is readily bioavailable. Oral absorption in calves was estimated at 1–11%, depending on the age. In humans up to 3% of an oral dose was recovered in the urine, indicating low absorption. In cows and ewes, 45–55% of the neomycin present in blood was bound to plasma proteins, and the remainder was present in non-ionized form and was distributed to the extracellular fluid. Neomycin is mainly excreted unchanged in the faeces after oral administration and in the urine after parenteral administration.

Single oral doses of neomycin were slightly toxic (LD_{50} = approximately 2250 mg per kg of body weight) in mice, whereas single intravenous doses were highly toxic ($LD_{50} \leq 100$ mg per kg of body weight).

Nephrotoxic effects were observed in mice and guinea-pigs following repeated subcutaneous administration of 30–300 mg of neomycin per kg of body weight per day and 10–60 mg of neomycin sulfate per kg of body weight per day, respectively. Similar effects were observed in dogs after repeated intramuscular administration of 24–96 mg of neomycin per kg of body weight per day. No kidney damage was observed in dogs given 100 mg per kg of body weight per day orally for 6 weeks. Ototoxicity was observed after repeated parenteral administration of neomycin at dose levels of 25–150 mg per kg of body weight per day in guinea-pigs and 20–80 mg per kg of body weight per day in cats. No ototoxic effects were observed in guinea-pigs dosed orally with up to 10 mg of neomycin sulfate per kg of body weight per day for 90 days. Auditory function was not affected in cats administered neomycin orally at 6.25, 12.5 or 25 mg per kg of body weight per day for 1 year; however, histopathological examination revealed changes in the organ of Corti at all dose levels.

The Committee concluded that, although ototoxicity was observed in the 1-year study in cats at the lowest dose tested (6.25 mg per kg of body weight per day), this study was inadequate for the safety evaluation of neomycin because of serious shortcomings in the histological technique and the absence of a clear dose-related effect. However, the Committee accepted the NOEL of 10 mg of neomycin sulfate per kg of body weight per day (equivalent to 6 mg of neomycin per kg of body weight per day) for ototoxicity from the study in guinea-pigs.

Only a limited number of mutagenicity studies were available, which had been poorly performed. The available *in vitro* genotoxicity tests indicated that neomycin causes chromosomal aberrations.

Tumour incidences were not increased in a 2-year toxicity and carcinogenicity study in which rats were administered neomycin orally at dose levels of up to 25 mg per kg of body weight per day. In the highest-dose males only a slight, but statistically insignificant, impairment of hearing was observed. Because the Committee regarded this effect as treatment-related, the NOEL was 12.5 mg per kg of body weight per day.

In a multi-generation reproductive toxicity study in rats in which neomycin was administered orally, no effects on reproductive parameters were observed at dose levels of up to 25 mg per kg of body weight per day, which was the highest dose used. A teratogenicity study with an unconventional protocol was conducted in the second generation (F_{2b}) female rats from the reproductive toxicity study. Neomycin was administered in the feed at 6.25, 12.5 or 25 mg per kg of body weight per day from days 0–6 and 16–20 of gestation; from days 6–15 of gestation, dose levels were raised to 62.5, 125 or 250 mg per kg of body weight per day. No malformations, fetotoxicity or maternal toxicity were observed.

Hypersensitivity reactions of the skin have been observed in humans following therapeutic treatment with neomycin. In addition, nephrotoxic and ototoxic effects have been observed after oral therapeutic use of neomycin.

From several *in vitro* microbiological studies with different bacteria, mostly isolated from humans, an MIC_{50} value of 64 µg/ml was derived for the most relevant sensitive species (*Escherichia coli* and *Lactobacillus* spp.) under conditions of high inoculum density. In germ-free mice inoculated with human gut flora, the NOEL for antibacterial activity was 125 mg per kg of body weight per day. Studies on the effect of neomycin on human gut flora in patients revealed effects at oral doses of 30 mg per kg of body weight per day and above.

Using the formula developed at the thirty-eighth meeting of the Committee (Annex 1, reference *97*), the Committee calculated a hypothetical temporary ADI based on antimicrobial activity as follows:

$$\text{Upper limit of hypothetical temporary ADI} = \frac{\text{Concentration without effect on human gut flora (µg/ml)} \times \text{Daily faecal bolus (g)}}{\text{Fraction of oral dose bioavailable} \times \text{Safety factor} \times \text{Weight of human (60 kg)}}$$

$$= \frac{64 \times 150}{1 \times 1 \times 60}$$

$$= 160 \text{ µg per kg of body weight}$$

It took the following factors into account:

- Factors to account for the range of MICs needed to account for sensitive bacteria, anaerobic environment, bacterial density and pH: the MIC_{50} value of 64 µg/ml was measured in the most relevant sensitive species under conditions of high inoculum density. No adjustment was deemed necessary.
- Availability: the Committee concluded that the experimental data were inadequate to correct for inactivation of neomycin as a result of binding to gut contents. It therefore took a conservative approach, assuming that the availability of ingested neomycin to organisms in the gastrointestinal tract was 100%.
- Variability among exposed individuals: a substantial amount of MIC data covering a variety of organisms, including anaerobes isolated from the human gut, was available. In addition, the Committee considered that the applied safety factor for the availability of neomycin to the gut flora was conservative. It therefore adopted a safety factor of 1.

In reviewing the available toxicological and antimicrobial data and in considering the hypothetical temporary ADI based on antimicrobial activity, the Committee concluded that the toxicological data provided the most appropriate end-point for the evaluation of neomycin.

Only a limited set of genotoxicity tests was available, with gene mutation studies in eukaryotic cells being absent. The available data indicated that neomycin causes chromosomal aberrations. However, the Committee noted that the long-term study in rats did not provide evidence for a carcinogenic potential of neomycin.

In view of the deficiencies in the genotoxicity data, the Committee established a temporary ADI of 0–30 µg per kg of body weight for neomycin, based on the NOEL for ototoxicity in the guinea-pig and a safety factor of 200.

Residue data

Neomycin has been used for more than 40 years as a human therapeutic agent for bacterial gastrointestinal infections. Neomycin sulfate has been used worldwide for over 35 years for treating bacterial gastrointestinal infections in cattle, sheep, goats, swine and poultry. It is also employed in the treatment of mastitis. Neomycin sulfate is available in various formulations, including premixes (for administration in the feed), water-soluble preparations and preparations for intramammary infusion.

Neomycin sulfate is used at dose levels of 10–20 mg per kg of body weight in cattle (150–350 mg per quarter when administered by intramammary infusion), 10 mg per kg of body weight in sheep, 10–15 mg per kg of body weight in pigs and 10–30 mg per kg of body weight in poultry. The duration of treatment with neomycin sulfate is 3–10 days for poultry and up to 14 days for larger animals.

Absorption of neomycin is poor (3–10%) from the intestinal tract in humans and animals and low from the udder. Absorbed neomycin accumulates in the kidneys and, to a lesser extent, the liver. It is not metabolized except by phosphorylation, adenylation and acetylation in the digestive tract; absorbed neomycin remains as the parent compound. A study in calves given [^{14}C]neomycin supports these conclusions except in very young animals (3–5 days of age). After oral administration of neomycin, over 90% of the dose is excreted in the faeces. The remainder of the dose is excreted in the urine. After intramammary administration, neomycin appears to be absorbed to a small extent in lactating dairy cows since neomycin residues were detected in the kidneys for up to 14 days after dosing.

Numerous studies were available in which neomycin was given to farm animals at various dose levels and times, primarily by the oral route. The Committee focused on the studies using the water-soluble formulations, because it considered that the concentrations of residues in the edible tissues would be highest in these studies. The Committee also reviewed residue studies in cattle, dairy cows, sheep, goats, pigs, chickens (broilers and laying hens), turkeys and ducks. At 0 hours after oral dosing, residue levels in the kidney tissue were 2.8 mg/kg in cattle, 2.2 mg/kg in pigs, 8.4 mg/kg in chickens, and 5.0 mg/kg in turkeys. In contrast, neomycin levels in milk and eggs were both below 0.2 mg/kg immediately after oral dosing. Residue levels in kidneys of sheep (at 1 day withdrawal) and goats (at 12 hours) were both 1.0 mg/kg; in ducks, the level was 0.89 mg/kg at 14 days withdrawal. After intramammary infusion of neomycin, the levels in milk were 0.22 mg/l and 0.07 mg/l at 48 hours and 72 hours withdrawal, respectively, while the level in kidney was below 5 mg/kg at 14 days withdrawal.

Methods of analysis
Adequate microbiological methods of analysis are available, which have quantification limits of 0.5 mg/kg in tissues and 0.2 mg/l in milk. HPLC and mass spectrometric methods are also available, with quantification limits of 0.1 mg/kg.

Maximum Residue Limits
Based on the residue studies and the temporary ADI of 0–30 µg per kg of body weight established by the Committee, the following temporary MRLs were recommended for cattle, sheep, goats, pigs, turkeys, ducks and chickens: kidney 5000 µg/kg, and muscle, liver and fat 500 µg/kg, expressed as parent drug. The temporary MRLs recommended for chicken eggs and cows' milk are 500 µg/kg and 500 µg/l respectively, expressed as the parent drug.

From the above temporary MRL values, the theoretical maximum daily intake of neomycin residues is 1275 µg, based on a daily food intake of

300 g of muscle, 100 g of liver, 50 g each of kidney and fat, 100 g of eggs and 1.5 l of milk (Annex 1, reference *85*). This is considerably less than the maximum ADI of 1800 μg of neomycin for a 60-kg person.

Results of the following studies are required for evaluation in 1996:

1. Gene mutation studies on neomycin, in particular in eukaryotic cells.
2. An *in vivo* study on chromosomal aberrations.

3.2.5 *Oxolinic acid*

Oxolinic acid had not previously been reviewed by the Committee. It is a quinolone antimicrobial agent that is active against Gram-negative organisms and is used as both a prophylactic and a therapeutic agent in aquaculture.

Although many more recently developed quinolone analogues are more effective, the relatively modest cost of oxolinic acid coupled with its satisfactory performance ensure its continued significant usage in aquaculture. Oxolinic acid is administered to fish and crustacea via incorporation into the feed at dose levels of 10–50 mg per kg of body weight.

Toxicological data

The Committee received toxicological data on oxolinic acid, including the results of acute and short-term toxicity studies, studies on absorption, distribution, reproductive toxicity and teratogenicity, and limited information on genotoxicity. However, because of serious shortcomings in the reporting and protocols, the Committee was unable to use these studies in its assessment. The Committee did not receive an evaluation report on oxolinic acid.

The Committee had access to published reports relating to oxolinic acid-induced juvenile arthropathy in dogs, carcinogenicity studies of oxolinic acid in rats and mice, and effects of oxolinic acid on clinical isolates and laboratory strains of bacteria.

Gough et al. (*5*) reported drug-induced arthropathy in young dogs following oral administration of oxolinic acid at 100 or 500 mg per kg of body weight per day for 14 days. Dogs in the high-dose group showed clinical signs of lameness, which disappeared upon exercise. Lameness was not observed in the low-dose group. Oxolinic acid induced degenerative changes in the articular cartilage and there was also a trend towards reduced serum alkaline phosphatase activity in both treated groups. A NOEL was not identified in this study.

Yamada et al. (*6*) performed a carcinogenicity study in which oxolinic acid was administered to rats at dose levels of up to 1000 mg/kg in the feed (equivalent to 40 mg per kg of body weight per day) for 104 weeks and to mice at dose levels of up to 500 mg/kg in the feed (equal to 58 mg per kg of body weight per day) for 78 weeks. Rats in the highest-dose group showed decreases in body-weight gain during the study. Increased incidences of tumours and hyperplasia of the Leydig cells and tubular atrophy of the testis were observed in males in the highest-dose group. In mice, decreased body-weight gain was observed in both sexes in the highest-dose group, but no preneoplastic or neoplastic lesions attributable to treatment occurred in either sex.

Izawa et al. (7) and Yamazaki et al. (8) investigated the effects of oxolinic acid on clinical isolates and laboratory strains of bacteria. From these studies, the concentration without antimicrobial effect on the most sensitive bacterial strain (*Escherichia coli*) was 0.25 mg/ml.

In view of the major deficiencies in the reporting and protocols of the toxicological studies available for evaluation, and as a clear NOEL in the arthropathy study in dogs could not be identified, the Committee was unable to establish an ADI.

Residue data

The extent of absorption following oral administration of oxolinic acid is only 10–30%, depending on the formulation of the feed. The remainder is released into the surrounding aquatic environment where it appears to be relatively stable. Very little is known about the distribution or degree of binding of oxolinic acid in different tissues and organs. There is little information on whether the drug is homogeneously distributed in the edible tissues of target species. In salmon, oxolinic acid is concentrated in the skin and bones and is depleted from these tissues at a much slower rate than from muscle or liver. The drug can be detected in significant concentrations in both the skin and bone at 180 days after treatment. In a study in which salmon were treated with the drug at 25 mg per kg of body weight for 10 days and then maintained in seawater at 6–14 °C, skin concentrations were 35 µg/kg after 180 days withdrawal.

The elimination of oxolinic acid from muscle and serum of fish has been extensively studied in a number of species. The elimination half-life depends on the species, and the temperature and salinity of the water. Studies in rainbow trout showed that the concentration of oxolinic acid residues in fish acclimatized to seawater decreased to undetectable levels in muscle after 3 days, whereas residue levels in the muscle of freshwater fish were still detectable after 10 days. The elimination half-life of oxolinic acid from freshwater trout was 6.1 days at 5 °C, 4.0 days at 10 °C and 1 day at 16 °C.

The withdrawal period recommended after dosing with oxolinic acid varies according to the fish species and the temperature and salinity of the water, and ranges from about 5 days for prawns raised in tropical salt water (28–32 °C) to more than 60 days for fish maintained at 8 °C in fresh water.

The metabolism of the drug in aquatic species has not been studied extensively and the fate of the drug is largely a matter of conjecture. One metabolic study of oxolinic acid in both seawater-acclimatized and freshwater trout indicated that glucuronidation of both oxolinic acid and products formed by the cleavage of the methylenedioxy ring of oxolinic acid constituted a major pathway of drug elimination. This was similar to the metabolism reported for mammals.

The extensive use of oxolinic acid is reflected in the numerous analytical methods available for its detection. Microbiological analytical methods have been developed but lack the sensitivity of chemical procedures. The majority of the chemical methods are HPLC procedures using either ultraviolet or fluorescence detection. Fluorescence methods are the most sensitive, with quantification limits of 0.5 µg/kg. A gas chromatography/mass spectrometry procedure suitable for confirmatory purposes has also been reported.

The Committee was not able to set MRLs for oxolinic acid because no ADI was established. No additional residue data were requested.

Before reviewing this compound again, the Committee would wish to have the following:

1. Resolution of the deficiencies in the protocols and reporting of the toxicological studies that were reviewed at the meeting.
2. Results of a study to identify a NOEL for arthropathy in dogs.
3. An assessment of the significance of the increased incidence of Leydig cell lesions observed in the recent carcinogenicity study in rats.
4. Either a detailed report, including individual animal data, of the recent carcinogenicity study in rats or genotoxicity studies to assess point mutation and chromosomal aberrations.

3.2.6 *Spiramycin*

Spiramycin had previously been evaluated at the twelfth and thirty-eighth meetings of the Committee (Annex 1, references *17* and *97*).

At its thirty-eighth meeting, the Committee established a temporary ADI of 0–5 µg per kg of body weight based on the estimated concentration without effect on the human gut flora, with the requirement of additional *in vivo* studies on the effects of spiramycin on the intestinal flora.

Toxicological and microbiological data
At its present meeting, the Committee considered data from new *in vivo* and *in vitro* studies on the effects of spiramycin on human gastrointestinal flora.

In an *in vivo* study in mice, a dilution of pooled faecal flora from healthy human volunteers was transferred anaerobically to germ-free mice. The animals were then treated with up to 200 mg of spiramycin per litre of drinking-water for 32 days. Increases in the number of resistant microorganisms were observed at 0.2 mg per litre of water, equivalent to 40 µg per kg of body weight per day. Although a quantitative end-point was identified, the Committee identified certain shortcomings in the study. There were large variations in the number of resistant coliforms and enterococci in the untreated control group and high populations of resistant microorganisms in all groups before spiramycin treatment. Moreover, only one concentration of spiramycin was employed for each bacterial group in the selective medium used to determine the total number of coliforms and enterococci and the number of resistant micro-organisms in the pooled faeces of mice.

The Committee also evaluated data from an *in vivo* study performed in chickens in which the effects of spiramycin on *Salmonella typhimurium*, *Escherichia coli* and several other microorganisms were studied. The Committee concluded, however, that this study was of little relevance for the microbiological evaluation of the effects of spiramycin on human gastrointestinal flora because the microorganisms investigated in the study were not of human origin.

Studies to determine MIC values for spiramycin were conducted using bacterial species isolated from healthy human volunteers. Dominant flora tested consisted of strictly anaerobic bacteria (10^9 bacteria/ml), while the subdominant flora included facultative aerobic and microaerophilic bacteria (10^7 bacteria/ml). A total of 110 strains were tested, all of which had MIC values of 1 µg/ml or above. These results confirmed those of the earlier studies evaluated at the thirty-eighth meeting of the Committee, performed on a limited number of strains. Taking into account the results of the studies already evaluated at the previous meetings, the Committee concluded that the new data provided further reassurance on the micro-biological safety of spiramycin.

At its thirty-eighth meeting, the Committee calculated a temporary ADI for spiramycin using the following formula:

$$\text{Upper limit of temporary ADI} = \frac{\text{Concentration without effect on human gut flora (µg/ml)} \times \text{Daily faecal bolus (g)}}{\text{Fraction of oral dose bioavailable} \times \text{Safety factor} \times \text{Weight of human (60 kg)}}$$

$$= \frac{1 \times 150}{0.05 \times 10 \times 60}$$

$$= 5 \text{ µg per kg of body weight}$$

At that time a safety factor of 10 was used to cover the variability between individuals of all extrapolated parameters.

In view of the additional reassurance provided by the new data, and as these studies covered a wide range of microorganisms, the Committee reconsidered the magnitude of the safety factor and concluded that a safety factor of 1 was appropriate. Taking into account the conservative margin of safety already provided by the parameters used in the formula, the Committee established an ADI of 0–50 µg per kg of body weight for spiramycin.

Residue data

At its thirty-eighth meeting, the Committee had requested data from radiometric studies on the concentrations of spiramycin and its metabolites as proportions of the total residue in edible tissues of cattle, pigs and poultry. As an alternative to the Committee's request, extensive studies were presented on residues of spiramycin and neospiramycin (the primary metabolite) in edible tissues of all three species, determined using HPLC and microbial inhibition assays with *Micrococcus luteus* ATCC 9341. These data provided useful information on the composition of spiramycin residues in edible tissues, but did not provide sufficient information to estimate the contribution of spiramycin and neospiramycin to total residues. Neospiramycin has an estimated antimicrobial activity of 88% compared to spiramycin.

In all residue studies in cattle, spiramycin and neospiramycin residues measured by HPLC accounted for about 100% of total antimicrobial activity in muscle tissue. In one example of such a study, in which cattle were given two intramuscular injections of approximately 32 mg/kg, 48 hours apart, residues of spiramycin and neospiramycin in liver tissue accounted for 93% of total antimicrobial activity at day 28 after dosing, and 67–100% (mean = 87%) of total antimicrobial activity at days 14, 21 and 35. In kidney tissue, these two residues accounted for approximately 100% (mean = 70%) of total antimicrobial activity at day 21, and 59–63% of total antimicrobial activity at days 14, 28 and 35. In fat, the parent drug and its primary metabolite accounted for 35–72% (mean = 54%) of total antimicrobial activity at days 28–35.

Similar studies were not reported for pigs, but data were available in chickens. In all residue studies in chickens, the concentrations of residues were significantly lower than in cattle and pigs at comparable post-treatment times. Because of the low residue concentrations in chickens, the ratios of spiramycin and neospiramycin to total antimicrobial activity were more approximate values than those reported in cattle. In long-term studies in which spiramycin was given in the feed at 110 mg/kg, residue concentrations in muscle, liver and kidney tissue were less than or equal to 0.015, 1.3 and 0.15 mg/kg, respectively. In a further study in which the drug was given in the drinking-water at 0.8 g/l for 3 days, residue concentrations were comparable. Spiramycin and neospiramycin residues accounted for approximately 100% of total antimicrobial activity in muscle, and 50% in liver, kidney, and fat tissue with skin. Polar metabolites may account for up to 50% of total antimicrobial activity.

In pigs, comparable studies were carried out only in liver tissue because of the complexity and amount of polar residues. In pigs treated orally with 50 mg per kg of body weight per day for 7 days, six quantifiable residues were identified and their structure was confirmed by mass spectrometry. The concentration of residues of parent drug was 0.4 mg/kg, while residue levels of spiramycin and neospiramycin adducts with L-cysteine were 10.5 mg/kg and 2.2 mg/kg, respectively.

Studies in pigs and poultry indicated that the metabolic pathway for spiramycin in these species was the same. Additional residue data from the plasma of cattle indicated that the metabolic pathway was similar to that in pigs and poultry. Spiramycin was metabolized to neospiramycin by hydrolysis of the mycarose side-chain, followed by conjugation of the aldehyde with L-cysteine to yield thiazolidinecarboxylic acid derivatives, tentatively identified as the major polar metabolites. The studies in pig liver were an important contribution to the metabolism studies because of the relatively high concentration of L-cysteine in this tissue. The Committee also took into account the studies on residue depletion reviewed at its thirty-eighth meeting.

Methods of analysis
An agar diffusion method using *Micrococcus luteus* ATCC 9341 as the test organism and an HPLC method were available for determining the concentrations of residues in the edible tissues and milk of cattle. The quantification limit of the agar diffusion method for spiramycin was 100 µg/kg in all tissues. Although the Committee considered that the agar diffusion method using *M. luteus* ATCC 9341 was suitable for measuring the antimicrobial activity of spiramycin residues, it may provide equivocal results. *M. luteus* has also been used for determining the antimicrobial activity of penicillins, streptomycin, erythromycin and neomycin. The HPLC method uses solvent extraction followed by reverse-phase liquid chromatography and ultraviolet detection. The quantification limits of the HPLC method for spiramycin were 30, 62.5, 30 and 47 µg/kg in muscle, liver, kidney and fat tissue, respectively. For neospiramycin, the limits of quantification in these tissues were 25, 50, 15 and 30 µg/kg respectively. For the agar diffusion method, the limit of quantification in milk was 62 µg/l. The Committee noted that a new HPLC method has been reported, which has a limit of quantification in milk of 13 µg/l for spiramycin and 6 µg/l for neospiramycin.

An agar diffusion method using *M. luteus* ATCC 9341 as the test organism was the only method available for residue analysis of pig tissue. The quantification limits for spiramycin and neospiramycin were 100 µg/kg in muscle, 300 µg/kg in liver, 150 µg/kg in kidney and 100 µg/kg in fat. A non-validated HPLC method was also used in some of the residue studies in pigs.

An HPLC method was available for determining the concentration of spiramycin and neospiramycin residues in poultry tissue. The limits of quantification in muscle, liver, kidney and fat are 50, 100, 200 and 75 μg /kg, respectively.

Maximum Residue Limits
Based on the ADI of 0–50 μg per kg of body weight established by the Committee using microbiological data, the permitted daily intake of spiramycin and its antimicrobially active residues would be 3000 μg for a 60-kg person.

In reaching its decision on MRLs, the Committee also took into account the available residue and metabolism data on spiramycin and neospiramycin, the percentage of total antimicrobial activity accounted for by these residues, and the limits of quantification for the HPLC and microbial methods. The Committee calculated the minimum residue levels that could be considered as a basis for MRL calculations using twice the limits of quantification for spiramycin and neospiramycin residues in cattle, pigs and chickens (see Table 6). These values were not adjusted to account for the percentage of antimicrobial activity represented by the sum of spiramycin and neospiramycin residues. In cattle, these two residues accounted for about 100% of the total antimicrobial activity in muscle, 85% in liver, 70% in kidney and 50% in fat. For pig tissues, the residues were determined by a validated microbial method. A validated chemical method for the determination of spiramycin and neospiramycin residues was not available; hence it was

Table 6
Minimum residue levels (μg/kg) that could be considered as a basis for MRL calculations for spiramycin in cattle, pigs and poultry[a]

Species	Analytical method	Minimum residue levels				
		Muscle	Liver	Kidney	Fat	Milk
Cattle	Agar diffusion using *M. luteus* ATCC 9341	200	200	200	200	124
	HPLC	60[b] 50[c]	124[b] 100[c]	60[b] 30[c]	94[b] 60[c]	26[b] 12[c]
Pigs	Agar diffusion using *M. luteus* ATCC 9341	200	600	300	200	NA
Poultry	HPLC	100[b] 100[c]	200[b] 200[c]	400[b] 400[c]	150[b] 150[c]	NA NA

NA: not applicable.
[a] Based on the quantification limits of the analytical methods, multiplied by a factor of 2. For the agar diffusion method, values refer to the sum of residues of spiramycin and neospiramycin.
[b] Values refer to spiramycin residues.
[c] Values refer to neospiramycin residues.

not possible to estimate the percentage of total antimicrobial activity accounted for by these residues. In chickens, these two residues accounted for about 100% of total antimicrobial activity in muscle, and 50% in liver, kidney and fat.

The recommended MRLs for spiramycin in cattle, pigs and chickens are shown in Table 7. For cattle and chickens, the MRLs are expressed as the sum of spiramycin and neospiramycin concentrations. For pigs, the MRLs are based on antimicrobial activity and are expressed as spiramycin equivalents; they are temporary for liver, kidney and fat, pending the availability of a validated chemical analytical method and the estimation of the percentage of antimicrobially active residues represented by the sum of spiramycin and neospiramycin in these tissues.

If these values are used for the MRLs, the theoretical maximum daily intake of antimicrobially active residues of spiramycin and neospiramycin from cattle and pigs would be less than that from chickens. The theoretical maximum daily intake of antimicrobially active residues from chickens is 250 µg, based on a daily food intake of 300 g of muscle, 100 g of liver, and 50 g each of kidney and fat. For cows' milk, the theoretical maximum daily intake of residues is 150 µg, based on a daily intake of 1.5 l.

The following information is required for evaluation in 1996:

1. A validated analytical method for determining the concentrations of spiramycin and neospiramycin in the edible tissues of pigs.
2. Residue data to estimate the percentage of total antimicrobial activity accounted for by spiramycin and neospiramycin in the liver, kidney and fat of pigs.

Table 7
Recommended MRLs for spiramycin (µg/kg) in cattle, pigs and chickens

Species	Recommended MRLs				
	Muscle	Liver	Kidney	Fat	Milk[a]
Cattle	100[b]	300[b]	200[b]	300[b]	100[b]
Pigs	200[c]	600[c, d]	300[c, d]	200[c, d]	NA
Chickens	200[b]	400[b]	800[b]	300[b]	NA

NA: not applicable.
[a] Expressed as µg/l.
[b] Expressed as the sum of the concentrations of spiramycin and neospiramycin.
[c] Expressed as spiramycin equivalents.
[d] Temporary MRL.

3.3 Glucocorticosteroid

3.3.1 *Dexamethasone*

Residue data

Dexamethasone had previously been evaluated at the forty-second meeting of the Committee (Annex 1, reference *110*), when an ADI of 0–0.015 µg/kg of body weight was established. At that time, new data were submitted by the sponsors of dexamethasone to facilitate the development of recommendations on MRLs for horses.

Depletion of dexamethasone residues in horses following a single intramuscular injection of 20 µg/kg was rapid. At 3 days after dosing, only kidney (0.57 µg/kg) and the injection site (1700 µg/kg) contained detectable residues of dexamethasone.

These data were in agreement with previous data for cattle and pigs and support recommendation of the same temporary MRLs for horses as those established at the forty-second meeting for cattle and pigs. Accordingly, the Committee recommended temporary MRLs for horses of 0.5 µg/kg for muscle, 2.5 µg/kg for liver and 0.5 µg/kg for kidney, expressed as parent drug.

3.4 Tranquillizing agent

3.4.1 *Azaperone*

Azaperone is a butyrophenone neuroleptic tranquillizer which had previously been evaluated at the thirty-eighth meeting of the Committee (Annex 1, reference *97*). At that time, an ADI was not established and the Committee requested the following information before reviewing the compound again:

1. Additional data from genotoxicity studies, which should include:
   (a) a study with the *Salmonella typhimurium* strains that were reported by one laboratory to be sensitive to azaperone and some of its metabolites; and
   (b) studies with cultured mammalian cells in which a variety of effects are investigated, including chromosomal aberrations and the induction of mutations.

   The results of these studies would determine whether further data are required.
2. Studies from which a NOEL for pharmacological effects in humans could be derived.
3. A justification for the protocol adopted in the reproduction study in rats that was submitted, and in particular for the very limited dosing regimen used in the females and the failure to dose the males.
4. Studies on the concentrations of residues of azaperone and azaperol in both muscle and fat of pigs treated with azaperone over a 3-day period.

Toxicological data

The information provided included data from a recent genotoxicity assay and an evaluation report that discussed all the toxicological and pharmacodynamic data that were considered to be relevant to the establishment of an ADI for azaperone.

The evaluation report stated that azaperone should not be considered carcinogenic since it is not genotoxic, it is not structurally similar to known carcinogens, and no unexpected adverse effects were demonstrated in the toxicity studies. However, there was no evidence available to support the claim that azaperone or its degradation products are not structurally similar to known carcinogens, and the Committee considered that such information should be provided.

The Committee reconsidered the results from the available genotoxicity assays. Conflicting results have been reported in two studies of azaperone, using the *Salmonella typhimurium* mutation assay. In one study, positive results were obtained in the presence of an exogenous metabolic activation system with azaperone and some of its metabolites. In contrast, no mutagenic effects were observed in the second and more thorough study. However, the metabolites were not tested in this study. The mutagenicity of azaperone and its metabolites in the *Salmonella* assay remains unresolved. A new study on cultured mouse lymphoma cells did not show mutagenic effects and the micronucleus and dominant lethal tests *in vivo* have shown no evidence of genotoxic activity. The Committee concluded that the weight of evidence suggests that azaperone has low potential for genetic damage.

In relation to the reproductive toxicity studies, the evaluation report stated that no adverse effects were found in the male genital tract in rats and thus a male fertility study was not performed. Although no histological changes were observed in the male reproductive tract, this is only one aspect in the assessment of reproductive performance. Therefore, the Committee concluded that effects on male fertility had not been adequately assessed and a study to assess reproduction and fertility in males was necessary.

Details were provided which confirmed the NOEL for sedation in humans of 30 µg per kg of body weight. However, the Committee was unwilling to use this study in establishing an ADI, since the observations were of a subjective nature and the experiment was poorly controlled. After reconsidering the pharmacological data, the Committee concluded that the NOEL of 630 µg per kg of body weight in a sensitive assay in the dog provided a more objective and appropriate measure of the pharmacological activity of azaperone.

The Committee considered that the pharmacological effects of azaperone were the most relevant for the determination of the ADI. A temporary ADI of 0–3 µg per kg of body weight was therefore established, based on the NOEL of 630 µg per kg of body weight for pharmacological activity in dogs and a safety factor of 200.

Residue data

At its thirty-eighth meeting (Annex 1, reference 97), the Committee requested studies on the concentrations of residues of azaperone and azaperol in both muscle and fat of pigs treated with azaperone over a 3-day period. Such data were provided by the sponsor for consideration at the present meeting. In addition, the sponsor provided information showing that the HPLC method using ultraviolet detection had been further improved and optimized for measuring residues of both azaperone and azaperol in tissues and plasma. The limit of quantification was 25 µg/kg in tissues and 5 µg/l in plasma.

Data submitted to the thirty-eighth meeting showed that azaperone was rapidly absorbed into the blood and was extensively and rapidly metabolized. The main route of excretion was via the urine in pigs and via the faeces in rats. One of the main metabolites found in rats and pigs was azaperol, which together with the parent drug, formed a major fraction of the residues. Many other metabolites were present, several of which were produced in both rats and pigs, although the relative quantities were different for the two species. These other metabolites did not possess significant neuroleptic activity when tested in rodents. The nature and bioavailability of bound residues were not addressed.

At its present meeting, the Committee considered a new residue-depletion study in pigs given a single intramuscular injection of 2 mg of azaperone per kg of body weight. After dosing, the residues in all edible tissues, excluding the injection site, depleted rapidly and were either not detectable or below 50 µg/kg at day 3. No residues were detected in these tissues at day 5 or day 7. Residues at the site of injection remained at significant levels for 5 days and were detected in one of four pigs at 7 days after dosing (see Table 8).

Table 8
Residue levels of azaperone and azaperol (mg/kg) at the injection site of pigs given a single dose of azaperone at 2 mg per kg of body weight intramuscularly[a]

Withdrawal time (days)	Residues	
	Azaperone	Azaperol
1	3–19	0.5–4
2	1–37	0.2–2
3	0.1–4	0.01–0.6
5	2–10	0.2–0.5
7	0.07	0.02

[a] For 7 days withdrawal time, values are for one animal; no residues were detectable in the other three pigs. All other values are for four animals.

Two residue-depletion studies in which pigs were given [³H]azaperone intramuscularly at dose rates of 1 or 4 mg per kg of body weight were submitted for consideration at the thirty-eighth meeting of the Committee. These studies indicated that residues were highest in kidney and liver. Approximately 5–20% of the total residues in these tissues were identified as parent drug or azaperol. A comparison of the data from the new residue-depletion study and from these two radiometric studies is shown in Table 9.

As suggested at the thirty-eighth meeting, both kidney and liver were possible target tissues. There were large variations in the ratio of the concentrations of azaperone to azaperol in different tissues and at different sampling times, and this made it almost impossible to use one of the compounds as the sole marker of the total residues. A more reliable marker of total residues was obtained if the sum of both compounds was used. The concentration of azaperone plus azaperol as a percentage of total residues was not known for the recommended dose (2 mg per kg of body weight); however, for the 4 mg per kg of body weight dose it was possible to calculate the percentage over a 3-day withdrawal time (see Table 10). The mean value for azaperone and azaperol as a percentage of total residues at all sampling times was 27% (range 6–115%) and at 72 hours after injection the mean value was 11%.

Maximum Residue Limits

Based on the temporary ADI of 0–3 µg per kg of body weight established by the Committee, the permitted daily intake of parent drug and its equivalents is 180 µg for a person weighing 60 kg.

Table 9
Residues of azaperone (µg/kg) in tissues of pigs sampled 24 hours after a single intramuscular injection of [³H]azaperone or unlabelled azaperone

Dose (mg per kg of body weight)	Residues[a]			
	Liver	Kidney	Muscle	Fat
1[b]	12	4	ND	ND
2[c]	<25	<25	<25	31–44[d]
4[b]	23	26	4	70

ND: not determined.
[a] For the lowest dose, values are for one animal; the values following administration of 2 and 4 mg per kg of body weight are for four and two animals respectively.
[b] [³H]Azaperone.
[c] Azaperone.
[d] Does not include one pig in which residues were not detected.

In reaching its decision on MRLs, the Committee took into account the following points:

- The temporary ADI was set on the basis of a pharmacological end-point.
- The sum of the parent drug and azaperol is a suitable residue marker and accounts for approximately 10% of the total residues in tissues. The remaining residues are not thought to possess significant neuroleptic potency and can therefore be discounted in calculating the MRLs.
- The limits of quantification for both azaperone and azaperol are 25 µg/kg in the tissues.
- The drug is indicated for use only in pigs.

The Committee recommended temporary MRLs in pigs of 60 µg/kg for muscle and fat, and 100 µg/kg for liver and kidney, expressed as the sum of the concentrations of azaperone and azaperol. If the recommended values are used for the MRLs and account is taken of the factors mentioned above, the theoretical maximum daily intake of residues of parent drug and azaperol is 36 µg, based on a daily food intake of 300 g of muscle, 100 g of liver, and 50 g each of kidney and fat.

The following information is required for evaluation in 1998:

1. Results of studies to determine the genotoxic potential of the metabolites of azaperone, which have been reported to be mutagenic in *Salmonella* spp.
2. Evidence to support the claim that azaperone or its degradation products are not structurally similar to known carcinogens.
3. Results of a study to assess the effects of azaperone on reproduction and fertility in male laboratory animals.

Table 10
Residues of azaperone plus azaperol as a percentage of total residues in tissues of pigs given a single dose of [³H]azaperone at 4 mg per kg of body weight intramuscularly [a]

Withdrawal time (hours)	Residues			
	Muscle	Liver	Kidney	Fat
2	51	20	14	115
24	15	11	10	72
48	14	10	18	35
72	11	9	6	19

[a] For 72 hours withdrawal time, the value for kidney is one animal; all other values are means for two animals.

4. Recommendations

1. Recommendations relating to specific veterinary drugs, including ADIs and MRLs, are given in section 3 and Annex 2.
2. In view of the large number of veterinary drugs requiring evaluation, meetings of the Joint FAO/WHO Expert Committee on Food Additives should be held annually for this purpose.

Acknowledgements

The Expert Committee wished to acknowledge the valuable contributions made to its work by Dr D. McGregor, Unit of Carcinogen Identification and Evaluation, International Agency for Research on Cancer, Lyon, France, and Dr Y. Yamada, Food Standards Officer, Joint FAO/WHO Food Standards Programme, Food and Nutrition Division, FAO, Rome, Italy.

References

1. *Residues of veterinary drugs in foods. Report of a Joint FAO/WHO Expert Consultation.* Rome, Food and Agriculture Organization of the United Nations, 1985 (FAO Food and Nutrition Paper, No. 32).

2. **Codex Alimentarius Commission.** *Report of the Eighth Session of the Codex Committee on Residues of Veterinary Drugs in Foods. Washington, DC, 7-10 June 1994.* Rome, Food and Agriculture Organization of the United Nations, 1994 (unpublished FAO document, ALINORM 95/31; available from FAO or WHO).

3. **Codex Alimentarius Commission.** *Report of the first Session of the Codex Committee on Residues of Veterinary Drugs in Foods. Washington, DC, 27-31 October 1986.* Rome, Food and Agriculture Organization of the United Nations, 1986 (unpublished FAO document, ALINORM 87/31; available from FAO or WHO).

4. **Commission of the European Communities.** The rules governing medicinal products in the European Community, Vol VI. In: *Part IV: Note for guidance on the application of the Annex of Directive 81/852/EEC with a view to the demonstration of the safety of a veterinary medicinal product.* Luxembourg, Office for Official Publications of the European Communities, 1991: 103-104.

5. **Gough A et al.** Juvenile canine drug-induced arthropathy: clinicopathological studies on articular lesions caused by oxolinic and pipemidic acids. *Toxicology and applied pharmacology,* 1979, **51**: 177-187.

6. **Yamada T et al.** Carcinogenicity studies of oxolinic acid in rats and mice. *Food and chemical toxicology,* 1994, **32**: 397-408.

7. **Izawa A et al.** Antibacterial activity of Miloxacin. *Antimicrobial agents and chemotherapy,* 1980, **18**: 37-40.

8. **Yamazaki T et al.** *In vitro* and *in vivo* antibacterial activity of a novel synthetic antimicrobial agent, 2-chloro-7-ethyl-4,7-dihydro-4-oxothieno-[2,3-b]pyridine-5-carboxylic acid. *Journal of Takeda research laboratories,* 1983, **42**: 297-307.

Annex 1
Reports and other documents resulting from previous meetings of the Joint FAO/WHO Expert Committee on Food Additives

1. *General principles governing the use of food additives* (First report of the Expert Committee). FAO Nutrition Meetings Report Series, No. 15, 1957; WHO Technical Report Series, No. 129, 1957 (out of print).

2. *Procedures for the testing of intentional food additives to establish their safety for use* (Second report of the Expert Committee). FAO Nutrition Meetings Report Series, No. 17, 1958; WHO Technical Report Series, No. 144, 1958 (out of print).

3. *Specifications for identity and purity of food additives (antimicrobial preservatives and antioxidants)* (Third report of the Expert Committee). These specifications were subsequently revised and published as *Specifications for identity and purity of food additives*, vol. I. *Antimicrobial preservatives and antioxidants*. Rome, Food and Agriculture Organization of the United Nations, 1962 (out of print).

4. *Specifications for identity and purity of food additives (food colours)* (Fourth report of the Expert Committee). These specifications were subsequently revised and published as *Specifications for identity and purity of food additives*, vol. II. *Food colours*. Rome, Food and Agriculture Organization of the United Nations, 1963 (out of print).

5. *Evaluation of the carcinogenic hazards of food additives* (Fifth report of the Expert Committee). FAO Nutrition Meetings Report Series, No. 29, 1961; WHO Technical Report Series, No. 220, 1961 (out of print).

6. *Evaluation of the toxicity of a number of antimicrobials and antioxidants* (Sixth report of the Expert Committee). FAO Nutrition Meetings Report Series, No. 31, 1962; WHO Technical Report Series, No. 228, 1962 (out of print).

7. *Specifications for the identity and purity of food additives and their toxicological evaluation: emulsifiers, stabilizers, bleaching and maturing agents* (Seventh report of the Expert Committee). FAO Nutrition Meetings Report Series, No. 35, 1964; WHO Technical Report Series, No. 281, 1964 (out of print).

8. *Specifications for the identity and purity of food additives and their toxicological evaluation: food colours and some antimicrobials and antioxidants* (Eighth report of the Expert Committee). FAO Nutrition Meetings Report Series, No. 38, 1965; WHO Technical Report Series, No. 309, 1965 (out of print).

9. *Specifications for identity and purity and toxicological evaluation of some antimicrobials and antioxidants.* FAO Nutrition Meetings Report Series, No. 38A, 1965; WHO/Food Add/24.65 (out of print).

10. *Specifications for identity and purity and toxicological evaluation of food colours.* FAO Nutrition Meetings Report Series, No. 38B, 1966; WHO/Food Add/66.25.

11. *Specifications for the identity and purity of food additives and their toxicological evaluation: some antimicrobials, antioxidants, emulsifiers, stabilizers, flour-treatment agents, acids, and bases* (Ninth report of the Expert Committee). FAO Nutrition Meetings Report Series, No. 40, 1966; WHO Technical Report Series, No. 339, 1966 (out of print).

12. *Toxicological evaluation of some antimicrobials, antioxidants, emulsifiers, stabilizers, flour-treatment agents, acids, and bases.* FAO Nutrition Meetings Report Series, No. 40A, B, C, 1967; WHO/Food Add/67.29.

13. *Specifications for the identity and purity of food additives and their toxicological evaluation: some emulsifiers and stabilizers and certain other substances* (Tenth report of the Expert Committee). FAO Nutrition Meetings Report Series, No. 43, 1967; WHO Technical Report Series, No. 373, 1967.

14. *Specifications for the identity and purity of food additives and their toxicological evaluation: some flavouring substances and non-nutritive sweetening agents* (Eleventh report of the Expert Committee). FAO Nutrition Meetings Report Series, No. 44, 1968; WHO Technical Report Series, No. 383, 1968.

15. *Toxicological evaluation of some flavouring substances and non-nutritive sweetening agents.* FAO Nutrition Meetings Report Series, No. 44A, 1968; WHO/Food Add/68.33.

16. *Specifications and criteria for identity and purity of some flavouring substances and non-nutritive sweetening agents.* FAO Nutrition Meetings Report Series, No. 44B, 1969; WHO/Food Add/69.31.

17. *Specifications for the identity and purity of food additives and their toxicological evaluation: some antibiotics* (Twelfth report of the Expert Committee). FAO Nutrition Meetings Report Series, No. 45, 1969; WHO Technical Report Series, No. 430, 1969.

18. *Specifications for the identity and purity of some antibiotics.* FAO Nutrition Meetings Report Series, No. 45A, 1969; WHO/Food Add/69.34.

19. *Specifications for the identity and purity of food additives and their toxicological evaluation: some food colours, emulsifiers, stabilizers, anticaking agents, and certain other substances* (Thirteenth report of the Expert Committee). FAO Nutrition Meetings Report Series, No. 46, 1970; WHO Technical Report Series, No. 445, 1970.

20. *Toxicological evaluation of some food colours, emulsifiers, stabilizers, anticaking agents, and certain other substances.* FAO Nutrition Meetings Report Series, No. 46A, 1970; WHO/Food Add/70.36.

21. *Specifications for the identity and purity of some food colours, emulsifiers, stabilizers, anticaking agents, and certain other food additives.* FAO Nutrition Meetings Report Series, No. 46B, 1970; WHO/Food Add/70.37.

22. *Evaluation of food additives: specifications for the identity and purity of food additives and their toxicological evaluation: some extraction solvents and certain other substances; and a review of the technological efficacy of some antimicrobial agents* (Fourteenth report of the Expert Committee). FAO Nutrition Meetings Report Series, No. 48, 1971; WHO Technical Report Series, No. 462, 1971.

23. *Toxicological evaluation of some extraction solvents and certain other substances.* FAO Nutrition Meetings Report Series, No. 48A, 1971; WHO/Food Add/70.39.

24. *Specifications for the identity and purity of some extraction solvents and certain other substances.* FAO Nutrition Meetings Report Series, No. 48B, 1971; WHO/Food Add/70.40.

25. *A review of the technological efficacy of some antimicrobial agents.* FAO Nutrition Meetings Report Series, No. 48C, 1971; WHO/Food Add/70.41.

26. *Evaluation of food additives: some enzymes, modified starches, and certain other substances: toxicological evaluations and specifications and a review of the technological efficacy of some antioxidants* (Fifteenth report of the Expert Committee). FAO Nutrition Meetings Report Series, No. 50, 1972; WHO Technical Report Series, No. 488, 1972.

27. *Toxicological evaluation of some enzymes, modified starches, and certain other substances.* FAO Nutrition Meetings Report Series, No. 50A, 1972; WHO Food Additives Series, No. 1, 1972.

28. *Specifications for the identity and purity of some enzymes and certain other substances.* FAO Nutrition Meetings Report Series, No. 50B, 1972; WHO Food Additives Series, No. 2, 1972.

29. *A review of the technological efficacy of some antioxidants and synergists.* FAO Nutrition Meetings Report Series, No. 50C, 1972; WHO Food Additives Series, No. 3, 1972.

30. *Evaluation of certain food additives and the contaminants mercury, lead and cadmium* (Sixteenth report of the Expert Committee). FAO Nutrition Meetings Report Series, No. 51, 1972; WHO Technical Report Series, No. 505, 1972, and corrigendum.

31. *Evaluation of mercury, lead, cadmium, and the food additives amaranth, diethylpyrocarbonate, and octyl gallate.* FAO Nutrition Meetings Report Series, No. 51A, 1972; WHO Food Additives Series, No. 4, 1972.

32. *Toxicological evaluation of certain food additives with a review of general principles and of specifications* (Seventeenth report of the Expert Committee). FAO Nutrition Meetings Report Series, No. 53, 1974; WHO Technical Report Series, No. 539, 1974, and corrigendum (out of print).

33. *Toxicological evaluation of certain food additives including anticaking agents, antimicrobials, antioxidants, emulsifiers, and thickening agents.* FAO Nutrition Meetings Report Series, No. 53A, 1974; WHO Food Additives Series, No. 5, 1974.

34. *Specifications for identity and purity of thickening agents, anticaking agents, antimicrobials, antioxidants and emulsifiers.* FAO Food and Nutrition Paper, No. 4, 1978.

35. *Evaluation of certain food additives* (Eighteenth report of the Expert Committee). FAO Nutrition Meetings Report Series, No. 54, 1974; WHO Technical Report Series, No. 557, 1974, and corrigendum.

36. *Toxicological evaluation of some food colours, enzymes, flavour enhancers, thickening agents, and certain other food additives.* FAO Nutrition Meetings Report Series, No. 54A, 1975; WHO Food Additives Series, No. 6, 1975.

37. *Specifications for the identity and purity of some food colours, flavour enhancers, thickening agents, and certain food additives.* FAO Nutrition Meetings Report Series, No. 54B, 1975; WHO Food Additives Series, No. 7, 1975.

38. *Evaluation of certain food additives: some food colours, thickening agents, smoke condensates, and certain other substances* (Nineteenth report of the Expert Committee). FAO Nutrition Meetings Report Series, No. 55, 1975; WHO Technical Report Series, No. 576, 1975.

39. *Toxicological evaluation of some food colours, thickening agents, and certain other substances.* FAO Nutrition Meetings Report Series, No. 55A, 1975; WHO Food Additives Series, No. 8, 1975.

40. *Specifications for the identity and purity of certain food additives.* FAO Nutrition Meetings Report Series, No. 55B, 1976; WHO Food Additives Series, No. 9, 1976.

41. *Evaluation of certain food additives* (Twentieth report of the Expert Committee). FAO Food and Nutrition Series, No. 1, 1976; WHO Technical Report Series, No. 599, 1976.

42. *Toxicological evaluation of certain food additives.* WHO Food Additives Series, No. 10, 1976.

43. *Specifications for the identity and purity of some food additives.* FAO Food and Nutrition Series, No. 1B, 1977; WHO Food Additives Series, No. 11, 1977.

44. *Evaluation of certain food additives* (Twenty-first report of the Joint FAO/WHO Expert Committee on Food Additives). WHO Technical Report Series, No. 617, 1978.

45. *Summary of toxicological data of certain food additives.* WHO Food Additives Series, No. 12, 1977.

46. *Specifications for identity and purity of some food additives, including antioxidants, food colours, thickeners, and others.* FAO Nutrition Meetings Report Series, No. 57, 1977.

47. *Evaluation of certain food additives and contaminants* (Twenty-second report of the Joint FAO/WHO Expert Committee on Food Additives). WHO Technical Report Series, No. 631, 1978.

48. *Summary of toxicological data of certain food additives and contaminants.* WHO Food Additives Series, No. 13, 1978.

49. *Specifications for the identity and purity of certain food additives.* FAO Food and Nutrition Paper, No. 7, 1978.

50. *Evaluation of certain food additives* (Twenty-third report of the Joint FAO/WHO Expert Committee on Food Additives). WHO Technical Report Series, No. 648, 1980, and corrigenda.

51. *Toxicological evaluation of certain food additives.* WHO Food Additives Series, No. 14, 1980.

52. *Specifications for identity and purity of food colours, flavouring agents, and other food additives.* FAO Food and Nutrition Paper, No. 12, 1979.

53. *Evaluation of certain food additives* (Twenty-fourth report of the Joint FAO/WHO Expert Committee on Food Additives). WHO Technical Report Series, No. 653, 1980.

54. *Toxicological evaluation of certain food additives.* WHO Food Additives Series, No. 15, 1980.

55. *Specifications for identity and purity of food additives (sweetening agents, emulsifying agents, and other food additives).* FAO Food and Nutrition Paper, No. 17, 1980.

56. *Evaluation of certain food additives* (Twenty-fifth report of the Joint FAO/WHO Expert Committee on Food Additives). WHO Technical Report Series, No. 669, 1981.

57. *Toxicological evaluation of certain food additives.* WHO Food Additives Series, No. 16, 1981.

58. *Specifications for identity and purity of food additives (carrier solvents, emulsifiers and stabilizers, enzyme preparations, flavouring agents, food colours, sweetening agents, and other food additives).* FAO Food and Nutrition Paper, No. 19, 1981.

59. *Evaluation of certain food additives and contaminants* (Twenty-sixth report of the Joint FAO/WHO Expert Committee on Food Additives). WHO Technical Report Series, No. 683, 1982.

60. *Toxicological evaluation of certain food additives.* WHO Food Additives Series, No. 17, 1982.

61. *Specifications for the identity and purity of certain food additives.* FAO Food and Nutrition Paper, No. 25, 1982.

62. *Evaluation of certain food additives and contaminants* (Twenty-seventh report of the Joint FAO/WHO Expert Committee on Food Additives). WHO Technical Report Series, No. 696, 1983, and corrigenda.

63. *Toxicological evaluation of certain food additives and contaminants.* WHO Food Additives Series, No. 18, 1983.

64. *Specifications for the identity and purity of certain food additives.* FAO Food and Nutrition Paper, No. 28, 1983.

65. *Guide to specifications – General notices, general methods, identification tests, test solutions and other reference materials.* FAO Food and Nutrition Paper, No. 5, Rev. 1, 1983.

66. *Evaluation of certain food additives and contaminants* (Twenty-eighth report of the Joint FAO/WHO Expert Committee on Food Additives). WHO Technical Report Series, No. 710, 1984, and corrigendum.

67. *Toxicological evaluation of certain food additives and contaminants.* WHO Food Additives Series, No. 19, 1984.

68. *Specifications for the identity and purity of food colours.* FAO Food and Nutrition Paper, No. 31/1, 1984.

69. *Specifications for the identity and purity of food additives.* FAO Food and Nutrition Paper, No. 31/2, 1984.

70. *Evaluation of certain food additives and contaminants* (Twenty-ninth report of the Joint FAO/WHO Expert Committee on Food Additives). WHO Technical Report Series, No. 733, 1986, and corrigendum.

71. *Specifications for the identity and purity of certain food additives.* FAO Food and Nutrition Paper, No. 34, 1986.

72. *Toxicological evaluation of certain food additives and contaminants.* Cambridge, Cambridge University Press, 1987 (WHO Food Additives Series, No. 20).

73. *Evaluation of certain food additives and contaminants* (Thirtieth report of the Joint FAO/WHO Expert Committee on Food Additives). WHO Technical Report Series, No. 751, 1987.

74. *Toxicological evaluation of certain food additives and contaminants.* Cambridge, Cambridge University Press, 1987 (WHO Food Additives Series, No. 21).

75. *Specifications for the identity and purity of certain food additives.* FAO Food and Nutrition Paper, No. 37, 1986.

76. *Principles for the safety assessment of food additives and contaminants in food.* Geneva, World Health Organization, 1987 (WHO Environmental Health Criteria, No. 70).

77. *Evaluation of certain food additives and contaminants* (Thirty-first report of the Joint FAO/WHO Expert Committee on Food Additives). WHO Technical Report Series, No. 759, 1987, and corrigendum.

78. *Toxicological evaluation of certain food additives.* Cambridge, Cambridge University Press, 1988 (WHO Food Additives Series, No. 22).

79. *Specifications for the identity and purity of certain food additives.* FAO Food and Nutrition Paper, No. 38, 1988.

80. *Evaluation of certain veterinary drug residues in food* (Thirty-second report of the Joint FAO/WHO Expert Committee on Food Additives). WHO Technical Report Series, No. 763, 1988.

81. *Toxicological evaluation of certain veterinary drug residues in food.* Cambridge, Cambridge University Press, 1988 (WHO Food Additives Series, No. 23).

82. *Residues of some veterinary drugs in animals and foods.* FAO Food and Nutrition Paper, No. 41, 1988.

83. *Evaluation of certain food additives and contaminants* (Thirty-third report of the Joint FAO/WHO Expert Committee on Food Additives). WHO Technical Report Series, No. 776, 1989.

84. *Toxicological evaluation of certain food additives and contaminants.* Cambridge, Cambridge University Press, 1989 (WHO Food Additives Series, No. 24).

85. *Evaluation of certain veterinary drug residues in food* (Thirty-fourth report of the Joint FAO/WHO Expert Committee on Food Additives). WHO Technical Report Series, No. 788, 1989.

86. *Toxicological evaluation of certain veterinary drug residues in food.* WHO Food Additives Series, No. 25, 1990.

87. *Residues of some veterinary drugs in animals and foods.* FAO Food and Nutrition Paper, No. 41/2, 1990.

88. *Evaluation of certain food additives and contaminants* (Thirty-fifth report of the Joint FAO/WHO Expert Committee on Food Additives). WHO Technical Report Series, No. 789, 1990, and corrigenda.

89. *Toxicological evaluation of certain food additives and contaminants.* WHO Food Additives Series, No. 26, 1990.

90. *Specifications for the identity and purity of certain food additives.* FAO Food and Nutrition Paper, No. 49, 1990.

91. *Evaluation of certain veterinary drug residues in food* (Thirty-sixth report of the Joint FAO/WHO Expert Committee on Food Additives). WHO Technical Report Series, No. 799, 1990.

92. *Toxicological evaluation of certain veterinary drug residues in food.* WHO Food Additives Series, No. 27, 1991.

93. *Residues of some veterinary drugs in animals and foods.* FAO Food and Nutrition Paper, No. 41/3, 1991.

94. *Evaluation of certain food additives and contaminants* (Thirty-seventh report of the Joint FAO/WHO Expert Committee on Food Additives). WHO Technical Report Series, No. 806, 1991, and corrigenda.

95. *Toxicological evaluation of certain food additives and contaminants.* WHO Food Additives Series, No. 28, 1991.

96. *Compendium of food additive specifications (Joint FAO/WHO Expert Committee on Food Additives (JECFA)). Combined specifications from 1st through the 37th meetings, 1956–1990.* Rome, Food and Agriculture Organization of the United Nations, 1992 (2 volumes).

97. *Evaluation of certain veterinary drug residues in food* (Thirty-eighth report of the Joint FAO/WHO Expert Committee on Food Additives). WHO Technical Report Series, No. 815, 1991.

98. *Toxicological evaluation of certain veterinary drug residues in food.* WHO Food Additives Series, No. 29, 1992.

99. *Residues of some veterinary drugs in animals and foods.* FAO Food and Nutrition Paper, No. 41/4, 1991.

100. *Guide to specifications – General notices, general analytical techniques, identification tests, test solutions, and other reference materials.* FAO Food and Nutrition Paper, No. 5, Rev. 2, 1991.

101. *Evaluation of certain food additives and naturally occurring toxicants* (Thirty-ninth report of the Joint FAO/WHO Expert Committee on Food Additives). WHO Technical Report Series, No. 828, 1992.

102. *Toxicological evaluation of certain food additives and naturally occurring toxicants.* WHO Food Additives Series, No. 30, 1993.

103. *Compendium of food additive specifications, Addendum 1 (Joint FAO/WHO Expert Committee on Food Additives (JECFA)).* FAO Food and Nutrition Paper, No. 52, 1992.

104. *Evaluation of certain veterinary drug residues in food* (Fortieth report of the Joint FAO/WHO Expert Committee on Food Additives). WHO Technical Report Series, No. 832, 1993.

105. *Toxicological evaluation of certain veterinary drug residues in food.* WHO Food Additives Series, No. 31, 1993.

106. *Residues of some veterinary drugs in animals and foods.* FAO Food and Nutrition Paper, No. 41/5, 1993.

107. *Evaluation of certain food additives and contaminants* (Forty-first report of the Joint FAO/WHO Expert Committee on Food Additives). WHO Technical Report Series, No. 837, 1993.

108. *Toxicological evaluation of certain food additives and contaminants.* WHO Food Additives Series, No. 32, 1993.

109. *Compendium of food additive specifications, addendum 2.* FAO Food and Nutrition Paper, No. 52, Add. 2, 1993.

110. *Evaluation of certain veterinary drug residues in food* (Forty-second report of the Joint FAO/WHO Expert Committee on Food Additives). WHO Technical Report Series, No. 851, 1995.

111. *Toxicological evaluation of certain veterinary drug residues in food.* WHO Food Additives Series, No. 33, 1994.

112. *Residues of some veterinary drugs in animals and foods.* FAO Food and Nutrition Paper, No. 41/6, 1994.

Annex 2
Recommendations on compounds on the agenda

Substance	Acceptable Daily Intake (ADI) and other toxico-logical recommendations	Recommended Maximum Residue Limit (MRL)
β-Adrenoceptor-blocking agent		
Carazolol	0–0.1 µg/kg of body weight	Muscle and fat/skin (pigs): 5 µg/kg[a, b] Liver and kidney (pigs): 25 µg/kg[a, b]
Antimicrobial agents		
Dihydrostreptomycin and streptomycin	0–30 µg/kg of body weight[c, d]	Muscle, liver and fat (cattle, sheep, pigs and chickens): 500 µg/kg[e, f] Kidney (cattle, sheep, pigs and chickens): 1000 µg/kg[e, f] Milk (cattle): 200 µg/l[e, f]
Enrofloxacin	0–0.6 µg/kg of body weight[c]	No MRLs recommended[g]
Gentamicin	0–4 µg/kg of body weight[c]	Muscle and fat (cattle and pigs): 100 µg/kg[a, e] Liver (cattle and pigs): 200 µg/kg[a, e] Kidney (cattle and pigs): 1000 µg/kg[a, e] Milk (cattle): 100 µg/l[a, e]
Neomycin	0–30 µg/kg of body weight[c]	Muscle, liver and fat (cattle, sheep, pigs, goats, turkeys, ducks and chickens): 500 µg/kg[a, h] Kidney (cattle, sheep, pigs, goats, turkeys, ducks and chickens): 5000 µg/kg[a, h] Eggs (chickens): 500 µg/kg[a, h] Milk (cattle): 500 µg/l[a, h]
Oxolinic acid	No ADI allocated[i]	No MRLs allocated[j]
Spiramycin	0–50 µg/kg of body weight	Muscle (cattle): 100 µg/kg[k] Muscle (pigs and chickens): 200 µg/kg[k] Liver (cattle): 300 µg/kg[k] Liver (pigs): 600 µg/kg[e, k] Liver (chickens): 400 µg/kg[k] Kidney (cattle): 200 µg/kg[k] Kidney (pigs): 300 µg/kg[e, k] Kidney (chickens): 800 µg/kg[k] Fat (cattle): 300 µg/kg[k] Fat (pigs): 200 µg/kg[e, k] Fat (chickens): 300 µg/kg[k] Milk (cattle): 100 µg/l[k]

Substance	Acceptable Daily Intake (ADI) and other toxico-logical recommendations	Recommended Maximum Residue Limit (MRL)
Glucocorticosteroid		
Dexamethasone	0–0.015 µg/kg of body weight[l]	Muscle and kidney (cattle, horses and pigs): 0.5 µg/kg[a, e, m] Liver (cattle, horses and pigs): 2.5 µg/kg[a, e, m] Milk (cattle): 0.3 µg/l[a, e, m]
Tranquillizing agent		
Azaperone	0–3 µg/kg of body weight[c]	Muscle and fat (pigs): 60 µg/kg[h, n] Liver and kidney (pigs): 100 µg/kg[h, n]

Notes to Annex 2

[a] Expressed as parent drug.

[b] The Committee noted that the concentration of carazolol at the injection site may exceed the ADI, which is based on the acute pharmacological effects of carazolol.

[c] Temporary acceptance (see Annex 3).

[d] Group temporary ADI for dihydrostreptomycin and streptomycin, individually or in combination.

[e] Temporary MRL (see Annex 3).

[f] Expressed as the sum of the concentrations of dihydrostreptomycin and streptomycin.

[g] The ADI for enrofloxacin is based on antimicrobial activity. MRLs were not recommended because the relationship between total antimicrobial activity and residues of enrofloxacin and ciprofloxacin could not be determined.

[h] Temporary MRLs were recommended because the ADI is temporary.

[i] An ADI could not be established for oxolinic acid because of major deficiencies in the reporting and protocols of the available studies and because a clear NOEL could not be identified for arthropathy in dogs.

[j] MRLs were not recommended for oxolinic acid because an ADI was not allocated.

[k] For cattle and chickens, MRLs are expressed as the sum of the concentrations of spiramycin and neospiramycin. MRLs for pig muscle and temporary MRLs for pig liver, kidney and fat are based on total antimicrobially active residues and expressed as spiramycin equivalents.

[l] The ADI for dexamethasone was established at the forty-second meeting of the Committee (Annex 1, reference *110*).

[m] The MRLs for dexamethasone in cattle and pigs were established at the forty-second meeting of the Committee (Annex 1, reference *110*).

[n] Expressed as the sum of the concentrations of azaperone and azaperol.

Annex 3
Further toxicological studies and other information required or desired

Antimicrobial agents

Dihydrostreptomycin and streptomycin

The following information is required for evaluation in 1997:

1. Information to assess the potential for effects on fertility and perinatal and postnatal toxicity.
2. An evaluation report or results of experimental studies on the metabolism of dihydrostreptomycin and streptomycin.
3. Data on residues of streptomycin and dihydrostreptomycin in eggs.
4. Results of studies to determine the relationship between the antimicrobial activity of the residues and their concentration, as measured by specific chemical methods.

Enrofloxacin

The following information is required for evaluation in 1997:

1. Detailed reports of the *in vitro* MIC investigations of enrofloxacin that were submitted for evaluation.
2. Information on the effects of enrofloxacin and ciprofloxacin on specific genera of microorganisms obtained from the human intestine.

In addition, the Committee required that the results of studies to determine the antimicrobial activity of the residues other than enrofloxacin and ciprofloxacin be submitted for review as soon as they become available.

Gentamicin

The following information is required for evaluation in 1997:

1. Results of studies on the effects of gentamicin on specific genera of microorganisms obtained from the human intestine.
2. Additional data to assist in the assessment of carcinogenic potential, which should include:

   (a) results of genotoxicity assays for gene mutations in mammalian cells and chromosomal aberrations *in vitro* and *in vivo*; and
   (b) details of an investigation on possible structural similarities between gentamicin and known carcinogens.

3. A validated chemical analytical method with a limit of quantification below the MRL recommended for milk.

Neomycin

Results of the following studies are required for evaluation in 1996:

1. Gene mutation studies on neomycin, in particular in eukaryotic cells.
2. An *in vivo* study on chromosomal aberrations.

Oxolinic acid

Before reviewing the compound again, the Committee would wish to have the following:

1. Resolution of the deficiencies in the protocols and reporting of the toxicological studies that were reviewed at the meeting.
2. Results of a study to identify a NOEL for arthropathy in dogs.
3. An assessment of the significance of the increased incidence of Leydig cell lesions observed in the recent carcinogenicity study in rats.
4. Either a detailed report, including individual animal data, of the recent carcinogenicity study in rats or genotoxicity studies to assess point mutation and chromosomal aberrations.

Spiramycin

The following information is required for evaluation in 1996:

1. A validated analytical method for determining the concentrations of spiramycin and neospiramycin in the edible tissues of pigs.
2. Residue data to estimate the percentage of total antimicrobial activity accounted for by spiramycin and neospiramycin in the liver, kidney and fat of pigs.

Tranquillizing agent

Azaperone

The following information is required for evaluation in 1998:

1. Results of studies to determine the genotoxic potential of the metabolites of azaperone, which have been reported to be mutagenic in *Salmonella* spp.
2. Evidence to support the claim that azaperone or its degradation products are not structurally similar to known carcinogens.
3. Results of a study to assess the effects of azaperone on reproduction and fertility in male laboratory animals.

World Health Organization Technical Report Series

* Prices in developing countries are 70% of those listed here.